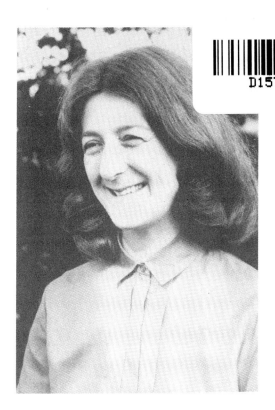

D1579972

Rowan Hillson, MD, MRCP is a Consultant Physician specialising in Diabetes and Endocrinology at Hillingdon Hospital,
Uxbridge. She has been involved in the treatment of Endocrine
disorders – thyroid disease being the most common – for many
years. Dr Hillson is very keen that people with thyroid disorders
understand their condition and treatment, and are aware of the
measures they can take to keep themselves healthy.

Also by Dr Rowan Hillson
and published in the
Positive Health Guide series

Diabetes: A Beyond Basics Guide
Diabetes Beyond 40
Diabetes: a Young Person's Guide
Diabetes: a New Guide

O P T I M A

THYROID DISORDERS

Rowan Hillson MD MRCP

Illustrated by Maggie Raynor

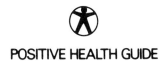

POSITIVE HEALTH GUIDE

© Rowan Hillson 1991

First published in 1991 by
Macdonald Optima

This edition published by
Optima in 1993

Reprinted 1994

British Library Cataloguing in Publication Data
Hillson, Rowan
   Thyroid.
   1. Man. Thyroid
   I. Title   II. Series
   612.44

   ISBN 0-356-18686-5

Optima
A Division of
Little Brown and Company (UK) LImited
Brettenham House
Lancaster Place
London WC2E 7EN

Typeset in Times by Solidus (Bristol) Limited
Printed in Great Britain by
J. W. Arrowsmith Ltd, Bristol

DEDICATION

For my grandparents

CONTENTS

ACKNOWLEDGEMENTS

I thank all the people with thyroid conditions who have shared their experience with me, and the physicians who kindled and maintained my interest in endocrinology. Without these patients and these professionals this book would not have been written.

I am also grateful to the following who contributed to the making and refining of this book: Jayne Booth, Michael Colston, Harriet Griffey, Kay and Rodney Hillson, Simon Hillson, Dai Thomas.

The table on page 54 is reproduced with kind permission of W.B. Saunders Company and is taken from *Textbook of Endocrinology* ed. Robert H. Williams, fifth edition, 1974.

The table on page 98 is reprinted from *Obesity*. A report of the Royal College of Physicians. *Journal of the Royal College of Physicians of London*, 1983, **17**, 1.

Every effort has been made to obtain permission to reproduce material in this book. Please contact the Publishers if there are any queries about copyright.

1

INTRODUCTION

Thyroid disorders are common, but they can be treated. About two in every 100 people have an underactive thyroid gland, and another two in every 100 have an overactive thyroid gland. But many more people have abnormalities of thyroid function without realising it, some of whom will come to need treatment.

This book is for people who have thyroid problems, whether overactivity or underactivity; for those who have been told they have minor thyroid abnormalities and for the families of people with thyroid disorders. Nurses and others who work with people who have thyroid trouble may also find it helpful.

The book is written in six sections: the first introduces the thyroid gland and how it works, the second considers the underactive thyroid gland and the third the overactive thyroid gland; the following sections discuss thyroid eye disorders and goitres; finally there is a section about looking after yourself and keeping fit. Throughout I have presented the problems from the perspective of the people who have them, starting with what they may notice wrong, followed by the visit to the doctor, diagnosis and treatment. Then I discuss the complications of the conditions and finally their causes.

I have used stories about people with thyroid disorders as examples. None of these people exist though – the names are all fictitious. But the stories do combine observations of many patients I have seen over the years.

One of the difficulties in writing information books for people with medical problems is that there are many ways of assessing, investigating and treating the condition; every doctor has his or her own way of managing the condition. Thyroid disorders are no different – there are many views on all aspects of the conditions. The fact that one doctor advises a different treatment from another does not necessarily mean that one is right and one is wrong – there are several ways of managing the same conditions, all of which are accepted and successful. I have tried to give an overview of the conditions and their management and an insight into some of the areas of controversy. But it is very important to remember that every person has his or her own unique version of the condition which needs individual attention from his or her doctor.

One of the aims of this book is to encourage you to think about your own condition and to ask yourself questions about what is happening in your body. Please turn to your doctor to help you answer such questions. He or she is the only one who knows all the details of your own very special case. It is also extremely important that you do not change your treatment without first discussing it with your doctor.

I believe that people should know the proper names for parts of their body, and that those who are unwell should know the medical terms for their condition and the tests and treatments relating to it. I have therefore used these terms throughout the book, but always with explanations. There is also a glossary at the end which explains most of the medical and scientific words used in the book (see pages 106–114).

2

THE THYROID GLAND

The thyroid gland lies in the neck. It is divided into two parts, a right and a left lobe, resting on either side of the Adam's apple. These lobes are linked by a narrow band of tissue called the isthmus. The thyroid gland is partly covered by the strap-like sternomastoid muscles that run from just below the angle of the jaw to the knobbles of the collarbones where they join the breastbone. You may be able to feel your thyroid – slip your

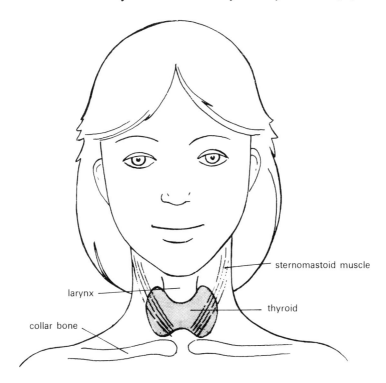

The thyroid gland in the neck.

fingers gently under the sternomastoid muscle and run them down on either side of the Adam's apple and the trachea (the windpipe); the thyroid is a softish tissue which goes up and down on swallowing.

In the unborn baby the thyroid gland starts life as a small piece of tissue at the back of the tongue, and gradually migrates down the neck to its adult site.

THYROID HORMONES

Like most body tissues the thyroid gland has a good blood supply, providing it with nutrients and removing waste substances. Because it is a gland, i.e. it produces secretions, these blood vessels also carry away the chemicals – the secretions – that the thyroid produces. These chemicals then travel in the bloodstream to all the parts of the body where they exert their effect. Such chemical messengers, produced by a small gland but acting throughout the body, are called hormones, and the glands that produce them – in this case the thyroid – are called endocrine glands. The hormones made by the thyroid are called thyroxine (T4 for short) and tri-iodothyronine (T3 for short).

If you look at the thyroid under a microscope you can see that it is made up of round balls of functioning tissue, called follicles. The follicles are set in non-functioning connective tissue through which the blood vessels run. Each follicle consists of a wall of follicular cells enclosing a gel-like centre called colloid. The follicular cells are the tiny factories which make thyroid hormones, and the colloid acts as a storage depot for thyroid hormones.

The raw materials for thyroid hormone manufacture are carried to the follicular cells by the bloodstream, the main raw material being iodine. We need about 100 to 200 micrograms of iodine a day, which we obtain from the food we eat. The iodine is transferred into the follicular cell from the bloodstream and chemically processed into thyroid hormone precursors – the chemicals from which thyroid hormones are made. At the same time, the follicular cell makes a special carrier substance called thyroglobulin. The iodine-containing hormone precursors are bound to the thyroglobulin, which oozes out of the follicular cell into the colloid. There the precursors undergo further chemical processing to produce T3 (which contains three iodine units) and T4 (which contains four iodine units). The mixtures of T3/T4/thyroglobulin are then

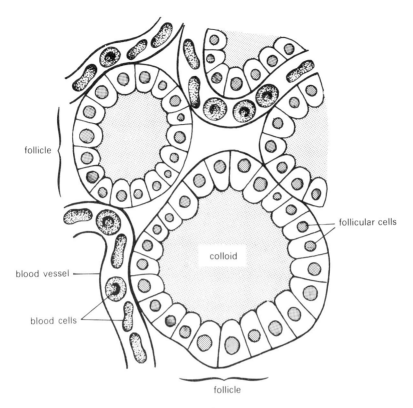

follicle

follicular cells

colloid

blood vessel

blood cells

follicle

Thyroid follicles as seen under a microscope.

stored in the colloid in the centre of the follicle.

When the thyroid hormones are needed the follicular cells take in tiny globules of colloid containing T3/T4/thyroglobulin. These are broken down inside the cells to liberate free T3 and free T4, which the cells then release – secrete – into the bloodstream. It it is this last stage in the process that constitutes the act of secretion (see diagram on next page).

CONTROLS OF THYROID HORMONE PRODUCTION

The thyroid gland is thus rather like a factory. Throughout the day the bloodstream delivers iodine and other raw materials and the thyroid makes them into T4 and T3 to be delivered to the rest of the body. But the thyroid gland itself has no control over the amount of T4 and T3 it makes; that is decided by the factory's head office – the pituitary gland, another endocrine gland.

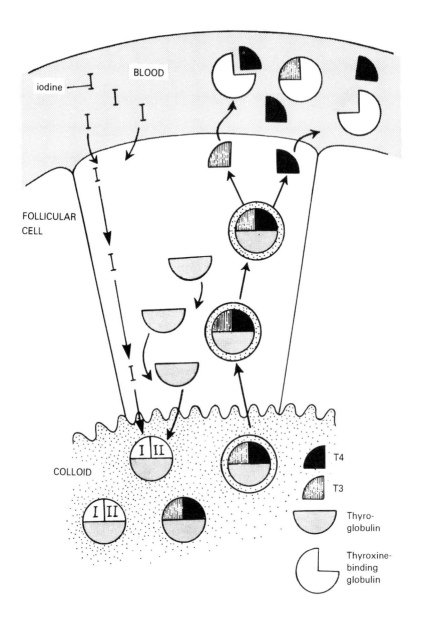

How thyroid hormone is manufactured in the follicular cell and released into the bloodstream.

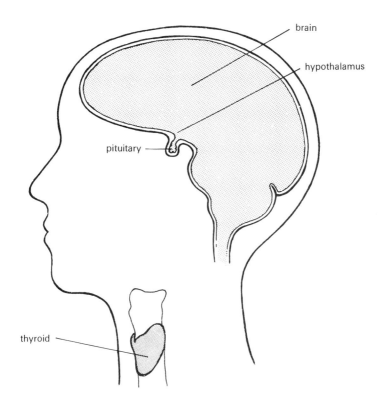

Position of thyroid in relation to the pituitary gland and hypothalamus.

The pituitary gland lies in a tiny bony chamber in the base of the skull. It is no bigger than a thumbnail in diameter, but is one of the most powerful organs in the body. Linked to the brain by a narrow stalk of tissue, the pituitary gland produces its own hormones which control the activities of most of the body's other endocrine glands. In the case of the thyroid gland the controlling hormone is called thyrotrophin or thyroid stimulating hormone (TSH for short). On thyroid cells there are specially-shaped places designed to receive TSH; these are called thyrotrophin or TSH receptors. When TSH links up with these receptors the thyroid gland is stimulated to produce and release T3 and T4: without TSH the thyroid does nothing.

The pituitary gland, in its head office capacity, usually works on a supply and demand basis. If more supplies of T3 and T4 are needed it produces more TSH so as to stimulate their production by the thyroid. If too much T3 and T4 appear in the bloodstream the pituitary shuts off TSH production, curtailing the overproduction of hormones by the thyroid.

7

The pituitary head office is, in its turn, told how much TSH to make by its managing director – the hypothalamus. The hypothalamus is a part of the brain which controls many sophisticated body functions, and is linked to the pituitary gland by the pituitary stalk. The hypothalamus releases a hormone called thyrotrophin-releasing hormone, or TRH, and it is this hormone that tells the pituitary gland what to do.

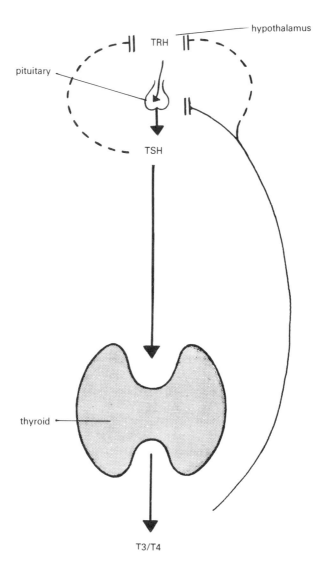

The relationship between the hypothalamus, pituitary and thyroid in the production of thyroid hormone.

TRANSPORT OF THYROID HORMONES

Ninety-nine per cent of the T3 and T4 travels around the bloodstream stuck to carrier proteins that transport them around until they are needed by the tissues. The main carrier protein is called thyroxine-binding globulin, but some T3 and T4 is also bound to a protein called albumin, and the rest is free in the blood.

With older methods of thyroid-hormone measurement this linkage with carrier proteins in the blood can sometimes lead to confusion; for instance, if there is a high blood protein level (such as can occur in women taking a contraceptive pill, for example) there can appear to be a high blood total T3 and total T4 level. Newer methods of analysis have resolved this problem by measuring free T3 and free T4 concentrations, so that the answer is not affected by blood protein level. There are about 9–24 picomols of free T4 per litre of blood and 5–10 picomols of free T3 per litre of blood, although each laboratory may quote slightly different normal ranges depending on their assay methods (methods of analysis) and other local factors. (A picomol is an extremely small unit of concentration, i.e. T3 and T4 are present in the bloodstream in very low concentrations.)

When the thyroid hormones reach the tissues which need them they separate from the carrier proteins and pass into the cells. T4 is not chemically active, however, and has to be converted to T3 before it can be used by the body. This conversion occurs in the heart, liver, kidney and other tissues, including the pituitary gland. In contrast the T3 made by the thyroid gland can be used straightaway.

WHAT DO THYROID HORMONES DO?

Thyroid hormones influence all the major body systems. They exert powerful effects on the tiny parts of cells called mitochondria in which many essential chemical processes occur, and are needed for other chemical reactions. They also influence the mechanisms by which fluids and chemicals enter and leave the cells.

In practical terms the effects of the thyroid hormones can best be seen by noting what goes wrong when a person makes too much or too little. This will be discussed in detail in subsequent chapters, but in general, the right amounts of thyroid hormones are essential for:

- Mental composure and alertness.
- Growth.
- Blood fat balance.
- Strong and steady heart function and blood circulation.
- Balancing the appetite, bowel function and body weight.
- Fluid balance in the body.
- Muscle strength.
- Ability to fight infections.

SUMMARY

- The thyroid gland is in the neck.
- It makes the thyroid hormones tri-iodothyronine, or T3, and thyroxine, or T4.
- The thyroid hormones are made in follicles by the follicular cells, and stored in the colloid of the follicles.
- Iodine is the main raw material for thyroid hormone manufacture.
- Thyroid hormone production is controlled by thyroid stimulating hormone, or TSH, which is produced by the pituitary gland in the head. TSH production is in turn controlled by the hypothalamus in the brain.
- T3 and T4 travel around the bloodstream linked with proteins.
- T4 is inactive and is converted to T3 for use by the tissues.
- Thyroid hormones influence all major body systems, the right amounts being essential for normal body functioning.

3

UNDERACTIVE THYROID – SYMPTOMS

There are two words used to describe an underactive thyroid – hypothyroidism (*hypo* means low) and myxoedema (spelt myxedema in America). Myxoedema (*myx* means mucus, while *oedema* means swelling) strictly speaking describes the firm non-watery swelling that sometimes occurs in the skin of people who have had untreated hypothyroidism for a long time; the term should be applied only to people with this problem, but long usage has made it more generally applicable. For this reason I will use it from now on in this book, simply because I want to avoid any confusion between the words hypothyroidism (underactive thyroid) and hyperthyroidism (overactive thyroid) – two words that look very similar on paper, but which are so very different in people.

SYMPTOMS OF AN UNDERACTIVE THYROID

A symptom is something you notice yourself. This chapter therefore considers the changes and feelings you may have noticed in yourself, one or more of which may have led you to seek medical help, if you have had an underactive thyroid. I have described the symptoms grouped together under the body system affected. This means that common and rare symptoms are listed together. The accompanying table will show you which symptoms are most frequently experienced.

Remember that in most people thyroid underactivity is detected early enough to prevent severe symptoms developing. Furthermore, no one person should expect to have all these symptoms. The symptoms of myxoedema are temporary and they get better with thyroid-hormone replacement treatment.

How common are the symptoms of myxoedema?

Symptom	Percentage of people with myxoedema who have the symptom
Weakness	99
Dry skin	97
Coarse skin	97
Lethargy	91
Slow speech	91
Swollen eyelids	90
Feeling cold	89
Decreased sweating	89
Cold skin	83
Thick tongue	82
Swollen face	79
Coarse hair	76
Pale skin	67
Forgetfulness	66
Constipation	61
Weight gain	59
Hair loss	57
Pale lips	57
Shortness of breath	55
Swollen hands/feet	55
Hoarse voice	52
Loss of appetite	45
Nervousness	35
Heavy periods	32
Palpitations	31
Deafness	30
Chest pain	25

GENERAL APPEARANCE

Dry skin, dry hair and brittle nails   The skin gradually loses its oils and starts to flake. Women may notice this before men; for example you may find that you need more moisturiser on your face. Your hands become dry and the skin becomes rather dull and lacklustre. The dry skin may be itchy, and you may notice thickened pads over the knees and elbows. You may not sweat as much as usual, which in turn contributes to your dry skin.

Your hair also becomes drier, and may start to fall out, so that some people who have had unrecognized myxoedema for a long time can develop very thin hair. Furthermore the hair becomes brittle and harder to control. Hair also grows more slowly than usual, and therefore you may find that you need to shave less often and visit the hairdresser or barber less frequently. Your eyebrows may thin out as well.

Your nails may become pale or white, grow slowly and break easily.

Sallow complexion You may develop a sallow complexion – the skin colour becomes paler and slightly yellowish in general, but the cheeks may become obviously pink or even red. This 'strawberries and cream' complexion is supposedly classical of myxoedema. The yellowness is due to a combination of anaemia and excess carotene in the blood (carotene is an orange-coloured precursor of vitamin A, and myxoedema interferes with its processing in the body). The change in complexion and the very dry skin may lead your beautician to suggest a visit to your doctor.

With myxoedema, even if you have a normal blood count your skin may look pale. However it is not uncommon for people with myxoedema to become anaemic as well, which can make you look very pale. The anaemia is rarely severe, though.

Weight gain Your weight may increase gradually over months, or even years, for the onset of myxoedema is insidious. You may not be eating any more than usual, or perhaps you are even eating less, but the pounds gradually accumulate (although large weight gains are uncommon), the increased weight being mainly fluid. Because of this your face may fill out

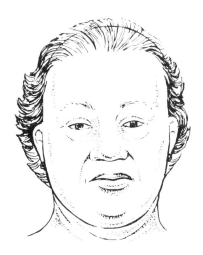

A person with severe myxoedema.

13

and your facial features become rather blurred – the classical appearance of myxoedema.

Thyroid hormone replacement (see Chapter 6) will reduce your weight to your pre-illness level. But I see many overweight people who are convinced that their obesity is due to a thyroid gland problem. Regretfully, this is rarely so – they are just eating too much for their body's current needs, so thyroid replacement treatment is not appropriate.

The weight gain is due to swelling; the classical feature of myxoedema. You may find that you have become somewhat puffy all over and that clothes, glasses, rings and shoes have become tight. Or you may have noticed swelling in the legs particularly; which by definition, is not supposed to pit, that is to dent when you prod it gently with your finger. But not every patient reads the textbooks. And some people with myxoedema do have pitting oedema. The swelling is due to leakage of protein-containing fluids out of the blood vessels and into the tissues, which in turn hold water in the tissues.

Slow healing and easy bruising You may notice that small cuts take longer to heal because the new skin grows slowly. Or you may be more prone to infections, which can take longer to resolve; this is because you need thyroid hormones for your body's defence mechanisms. Easy bruising is another symptom, due to fragility of the blood vessels.

BRAIN AND NERVOUS SYSTEM

Slowing down Slowing down is a very common symptom of myxoedema. As the levels of T3 and T4 fall, your brain gradually slows down. For example, you may notice that you are not doing as much each day as you used to; it may take longer to do jobs or plan things than before; you may think more slowly than you used to; you may be less likely to take the initiative, letting others think for you. Sometimes it is other people – your family or friends – who tell you that you have slowed down.

Tiredness, sleepiness, lack of energy Tiredness is another common, but rather vague, symptom. Lack of thyroid hormone may make you feel generally worn out; the day's work may take so much out of you that you have to have a rest as soon as you get home. Sometimes people with an underactive thyroid fall asleep very easily – at their desks or after lunch, for example. Or it becomes easy to nod off after dinner in the evenings.

These feelings of tiredness and lack of energy may also combine with the general slowing down.

Getting muddled   The brain needs thyroid hormone as much as any other part of the body, so if T3 and T4 levels are low the brain does not work quite as well as it should. This can show itself as minor forgetfulness, or getting muddled over your change when shopping; you may forget people's names or become absent-minded. Rarely, people develop more severe confusion. Children who have lacked thyroid hormone from birth may develop mental retardation or cretinism; early thyroxine treatment completely prevents this tragedy. Modern paediatrics has virtually abolished cretinism.

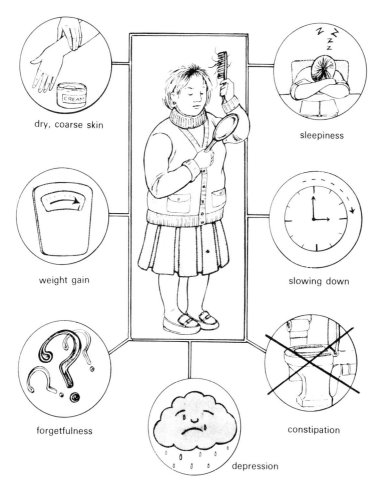

Symptoms of myxoedema.

Depression or other psychiatric symptoms Very rarely, people with myxoedema develop psychiatric symptoms. Sometimes they become depressed; in the old days, people with myxoedema were occasionally labelled as suffering from depression and given psychiatric treatment – as many of the symptoms of myxoedema mimic those of depression, one can understand why. Occasionally people with myxoedema may temporarily become very disturbed, perhaps believing that their family are trying to poison them, or become very aggressive. Because of this, I believe that every depressed or confused person should have his or her thyroid function checked as a matter of routine; the psychiatric symptoms associated with myxoedema can be completely cured by thyroid replacement therapy, thus obviating the need for psychiatric treatment in such cases.

Incoordination This is a rare symptom. The part of the brain which controls balance and coordination (the cerebellum) can be affected by severe myxoedema, leading to clumsiness, poor balance, with falls in elderly people, trembling hands when reaching out for things, and poor coordination. All these settle with treatment.

Numbness and tingling Quite often, people with myxoedema may feel numbness, tingling or pins and needles in their hands and feet. This is probably due to pressure on nerves caused by tissue swelling. In the hands, the median nerve can be squashed as it passes through the carpal tunnel at the wrist, causing numbness or tingling in the thumb and first two fingers.

Headaches, coma You may have more headaches than usual, which you will be aware of. And you may even suffer from unconsciousness, which you will not be aware of. Nowadays, fortunately, the latter, known as myxoedema coma, is very uncommon; it may occur in people with myxoedema who get very cold, have a severe infection or accident, or who are short of oxygen. Fits can rarely occur.

Eyes Eye trouble is more often associated with an overactive thyroid gland than an underactive one. However, people can swing from overactive to underactive, and this may affect any eye condition accompanying the initial overactivity (see Chapter 15 for details). In myxoedema the eyelids are often puffy and may be sticky in the morning, needing a lot of rubbing, which can cause soreness. Another cause of soreness due to rubbing is watery eyes or epiphora. Occasionally, night vision may be poor.

EAR, NOSE AND THROAT

Hearing   You may be troubled by slight deafness. Usually this simply means that the television sound needs to be turned up a little, although occasionally the hearing impairment is more of a nuisance. There is also a rare inherited condition, with symptoms of white streaks in the hair, underactive thyroid and more severe deafness (Pendred's syndrome).

Snoring   People with myxoedema often snore loudly; you are unlikely to notice this yourself, but your partner will. This, combined with falling asleep easily, can lead to some social embarrassment – in the theatre, for example. The increased tendency to snoring is probably due to a thickening of the tissues at the back of the throat. Your tongue may feel large in your mouth.

Hoarse voice   Thickening of the vocal cords may cause your voice to become husky. In a few people the voice becomes very hoarse and you sound as if you have a permanent sore throat. Sometimes the voice is deeper, especially in women, or a little slurred.

Swollen neck   You may also have a swollen neck caused by a swollen thyroid. This is called a goitre, and can occur in the presence of normal thyroid hormone levels, excess T3 and T4, or in people with myxoedema. See Chapter 16 for a detailed look at goitre.

DIGESTIVE SYSTEM

Poor appetite   You may lose your appetite. And it can be very puzzling for a person who is eating less than normal to find themselves putting on weight.

Constipation   In myxoedema your bowels slow down, like the rest of your body, and move faeces through the system at a slower rate. This can lead to very stubborn constipation. In a few elderly people, whose bowels have poor muscle tone to start with, the constipation can become so severe that medicines and pills are to no avail and the person develops bowel obstruction; they can start vomiting and become very ill. In this instance the person may be sent into hospital to see a surgeon, although it is rare for an operation to be needed – treatment of the myxoedema, fluids and enemas slowly resolve the problem.

HEART, CIRCULATION AND LUNGS

Cold intolerance Cold intolerance is a relatively specific symptom of thyroid underactivity. Room temperatures in which you previously felt comfortable are now too low, and you need extra fires or have to turn the thermostat to a higher setting. You start adding more and more clothes. At night you pile on extra blankets and still feel cold. 'I just can't get warm, doctor' is one of the commonest complaints of a person with myxoedema. Sometimes it happens so gradually that it is a relative who notices the problem first; they are sweating and taking off layers of clothes as you turn up the central heating. The cold intolerance is mainly due to sluggish circulation, for your heart pumps less often and less strongly if you have severe myxoedema. When thyroid hormone levels are low the body's chemical processes, or metabolism slow down, including those that break down the food we eat and covert it into the energy which powers body functions. These processes release heat as a byproduct, which helps to keep you warm, so if the metabolism is functioning at a reduced level, less heat is produced.

Cold hands and feet As the circulation slows down your hands and feet may become particularly cold.

Shortness of breath You may find yourself a little puffed on hills or going upstairs, although severe shortness of breath is rare. This may be due to several factors – fluid accumulation around the lungs, the slow heart rate and less strong heart beat, anaemia and excess weight.

Chest pain Chest pain may also occur, although this is not a symptom of the thyroid underactivity but of its consequences. Lack of T3 and T4 alters fat metabolism (see page 34) and this can lead to furring of the coronary arteries (coronary atherosclerosis) and reduction of blood supply to some of the heart muscle. This causes angina (see page 44) – pain in the chest on exercising, which is usually relieved by rest. Angina is rare in people with myxoedema – call your doctor immediately if you have chest pain.

18

Blackouts   These are an infrequent way for myxoedema to show itself. Like the rest of the body, the heart slows down and the pulse rate may become so slow that the heart stops briefly and then recovers again. This situation may require emergency treatment to help the heart keep beating steadily while thyroid replacement treatment is started. You should see your doctor immediately if you have a blackout.

BONES AND MUSCLES

Weak muscles and stiff joints   People with myxoedema often say that their muscles feel weak and stiff, and that they ache. As part of the general slowing up, your muscles may respond very slowly. In addition they may also be slow to return to normal after a movement, although few people notice this themselves. As a result it may be hard to do things as vigorously as usual; sportsmen may find a considerable fall in their performance. You may think you have arthritis, with stiff and aching joints. The joints only rarely become swollen, though.

Growing   Children with severe myxoedema do not grow properly. Fortunately, childhood myxoedema is uncommon nowadays.

SEXUAL FUNCTION

Period problems   Thyroid hormone lack can cause confusion in other hormone systems. For example, erratic sex hormone production can cause heavy and irregular periods.

Lack of interest in sex   You may be too tired for sex, and have a headache, but in addition the interference with sex hormones which occurs can reduce your libido or sexual drive, whether you are a man or a woman.

Infertility   If the sex hormones are confused, the ovum may not be released and then the woman cannot conceive; a man may make insufficient sperm. Rarely, a woman with untreated myxoedema may have a miscarriage. Thyroid hormone levels are measured routinely in infertility clinics, for underactivity is readily treatable, allowing a return to normal fertility.

SUMMARY

There are many symptoms of myxoedema, but no one has all of them. They include:

- Changes in appearance such as dry skin, sallow complexion, weight gain and swelling.
- Slowing down, tiredness, energy lack and other changes in thinking or behaviour.
- Ear, nose and throat symptoms include hoarseness and deafness.
- Constipation is a common digestive symptom.
- Cold intolerance is a classical symptom of myxoedema.
- Muscles may become weak, joints stiff and fingers numb.
- There may be problems with periods and sex life.

The symptoms all improve with thyroid hormone replacement treatment.

4

UNDERACTIVE THYROID – WHAT THE DOCTOR LOOKS FOR

All doctors are taught to record your story and to examine you in much the same way; this is so that they obtain all the information they need to help you every time. Of course, they will adjust the questions and examination to suit the condition, but if you understand how your doctor's mind works it will make it easier for you to explain matters and for him to assess you. Try jotting down information before you see the doctor so that you make sure you tell him everything you are worried about.

YOUR STORY

Your doctor will want to know why you have decided to come to see him/her and what symptoms have been worrying you most. Remember, symptoms are things you have noticed wrong with yourself or unusual feelings. So tell him the most worrying things first, and then the others. Tell him how it all began, from the time you last felt really well, and how it has progressed since then. It helps to know when each symptom started, when it stopped (or if you still have it), what brings it on, what makes it better or worse, and, most of all, exactly what the symptom consists of. For example, contrast 'I feel rather cold, doctor' with 'I always feel cold all over, doctor, even if other people are hot. My hands and feet are especially cold. I've turned the central heating up but I still need extra bedclothes. I first noticed it 4 months ago, but it's getting worse.'

Once you have told your story, the doctor may ask you some questions to clarify details and to gain further information about related symptoms.

Previous medical history

It is important to tell every new doctor you see about illnesses and operations you have had in the past, or conditions you still have, even if you cannot see how they might influence your current illness. For example, you may have nearly forgotten the bout of rheumatic fever you had 30 years ago when you were ten years old – surely that's got nothing to do with thyroid trouble. No, it hasn't, but your breathlessness and swollen ankles may be due to heart damage from rheumatic fever rather than fluid retention from myxoedema.

Have you ever had a thyroid operation? Or X-ray treatment to your neck? Have you ever had an overactive thyroid, and, if so, what treatment did you have for it? Did you ever have radioactive iodine treatment? Do you have diabetes or pernicious anaemia?

Family history

As you will see later (pages 46–7), thyroid disease runs in families. Does anyone in your family have an overactive thyroid or an underactive one? Did they in the past? Is there a family history of diabetes or pernicious anaemia?

Your job and lifestyle

Some parts of the country, for example, Derbyshire, are associated with iodine lack and goitre, so your doctor will be interested in where you live now and where you lived before.

Your job and responsibilities are unlikely to have included factors which cause thyroid disease, but it is important that your doctor understands what you do and what it entails mentally and physically. Also, are you responsible for other people's safety? Do you have to make rapid decisions or rely on strong muscles or finely balanced movements?

What sort of person are you? Are you usually the life and soul of the party, but have now slowed down and are a bit miserable because of myxoedema? Or have you always been a quiet, steady person, so that no one noticed you gradually become quieter and start to slow down?

Eating, drinking and smoking   As weight gain, despite loss of appetite, is often a symptom of thyroid underactivity, your doctor may want to know how much you usually eat and whether your eating pattern has changed. What sort of foods do you eat? For example, people who eat huge quantities of cabbage are supposed to be more likely to have thyroid swelling or goitres. Do you eat a lot of fatty foods? Your blood cholesterol level is likely to be high until your thyroid underactivity is treated. Drinking excessive alcohol or any smoking at all are both major health hazards, whatever your underlying illness, and smoking is especially hazardous in people with a high cholesterol level.

Drugs and medicines. Allergies   Do you take any drugs? By this I don't mean street drugs – although if you have ever taken these you should tell your doctor. I mean any kind of pills, tablets, potions, medicines, injections, unguents, herbal remedies, homoeopathic medicines you may be using. It includes medicines you have bought at the pharmacists, like aspirin or paracetamol. It is vitally important that you know what you are taking and that you make sure every doctor you see knows what you are taking. So often, people only tell a particular doctor about the medicines in which they think he is interested. So they will list their blood pressure pills to Dr Jones but omit to mention their heart pills ('I see Dr Brown for that'). Then they wonder why they feel poorly when Dr Jones prescribes new blood pressure pills (because the new pills do not mix with the heart pills). Some drugs, like aspirin, can interfere with thyroid function tests. And some herbal remedies may contain salicylates (the active ingredient of aspirin) or may contain large quantities of iodine – seaweed pills, for example.

Always tell your doctor if you think you have had a reaction to your medication. And if you have had such a reaction (an allergy or other unwanted effect) to any medication, make sure you know exactly what the proper name of the drug was and what it did to you. The name should be printed on the label of the bottle or on your prescription card. Check with your doctor. Write the name down and then tell every doctor you see what happened.

The rest of your body

Once the details of your story have been checked, the doctor may ask some apparently totally irrelevant questions. These so-called direct questions are to check that the rest of you is all right – your chest, digestive system, urinary system, and so on.

EXAMINATION – LOOKING FOR SIGNS

A sign is something your doctor finds when he examines you. For example, if you have myxoedema you may walk slowly into the room and sit down listlessly. Your handshake may be slow to grip and relax, and cold, and your 'Good afternoon' husky or hoarse. You may respond slowly to questions and it may take a long time to work out the answers. You may look sad or very sleepy. You are probably wearing thick sweaters and a coat, despite the warmth of the consulting room.

You may be overweight, and pale with a sallow complexion and sometimes pink/red cheeks. There may be yellow/white fatty deposits on your upper eyelids (called xanthelasmata) and white fatty rings (called corneal arcus) around the iris of the eye (the coloured bit). Your face, especially the eyelids, may be puffy. Other puffy areas might include the hands (especially the backs), and the tops of the feet. Your skin may look dry and flaky, with areas of thick dry skin on pressure points like the elbows and heels. You may have bruises. Your nails may be white, dry and broken and the hair thin and lacklustre. The outer third of the eyebrows may be thin or missing.

Your doctor will be able to observe all of these signs without touching you; indeed, they may be sufficient to make the diagnosis clinically.

Your skin may feel cold and dry to the touch. Anaemia may be diagnosed by looking at the pallor of the hands and the lower eyelids. The tongue may appear full. You may have an obvious thyroid swelling – or it may not be possible to feel the thyroid gland at all.

Heart, circulation and lungs

A slow pulse is characteristic of myxoedema (a slow pulse is called bradycardia). Your hands and feet may have reduced circulation, although the main pulses can be readily felt. Your blood pressure may be low or normal. In severe myxoedema the heart may be enlarged due to fluid around it – called pericardial effusion – but this is rare. If the heart has been severely weakened by lack of thyroid hormone there may be heart failure, with pitting swelling of feet and ankles.

The lungs   The lungs are rarely affected by myxoedema, but occasionally fluid surrounds them and this can be detected by your doctor, who will tap your chest with his fingers and listen to your breathing.

The abdomen

The abdomen often feels doughy and dry. Your internal organs will usually be normal, but your doctor may feel the fullness and lumpiness of your bowel if you have severe constipation. If the constipation has been very troublesome or caused you abdominal pain he may perform a rectal examination by gently inserting a lubricated gloved finger into the rectum. This does not hurt but is just slightly uncomfortable and may make you feel as if you want to open your bowels.

Some men may develop scrotal swelling if fluid accumulates there. This is called hydrocele and is not serious.

Nervous system including vision and hearing

Daytime vision is usually normal, unless thyroid eye disease has caused problems (see pages 89–93). But your hearing may be reduced; to check it your doctor may ask you to listen to a tuning fork. If you have complained of weak muscles he may test your strength, looking at each limb in turn. It is also important to check your tendon reflexes by tapping the elbows, wrists, knees and ankles with a small tendon hammer. Classically the reflex jerks relax slowly in myxoedema. A few hospitals have machines that you kneel beside which measure the relaxation time of the tendon reflex at the ankle.

If you have noticed numbness, pins and needles or tingling, the doctor will ask you exactly where the problem is, and may then touch the skin lightly with cotton wool or a clean pin to check sensation. Tapping over the carpal tunnel at the wrist can sometimes reproduce tingling, due to median nerve compression there. Another name for this is carpal tunnel syndrome (see page 16).

In the few people with myxoedema who have noticed balance or coordination problems, the doctor will probably check how well you can point to things and how dextrous your fingers are. He may also ask you to walk heel-to-toe to check your balance.

CASE HISTORY OF MYXOEDEMA

John Green is a 58-year-old taxi driver, and has lived in London all his life. This is his case history as written down by a doctor.

Patient complains of

- 'I'm tired all the time.'
- 'I keep falling asleep.'
- 'I feel the cold, even in summer.'

History of presenting complaint

For the past six months Mr Green has been excessively tired and fallen asleep readily, both at home and at work. Once he fell asleep in his cab while waiting in a traffic jam. Although previously a 'night-owl', he now goes to bed at 8pm. He feels exhausted all the time and has little energy. He has marked cold intolerance and wears extra clothes day and night. His hands and feet are particularly cold, and he now wears gloves for driving, although he never did so previously.

On direct questioning, Mr Green cannot concentrate and finds it hard to calculate the change for customers. He knows London well after 30 years taxi-driving but has recently got lost on several occasions. He has gained about five pounds in weight but thinks his appetite is normal. He has had increasing constipation for four months, opening his bowels once every three or four days, compared with daily before. The motions are hard but normal in colour. He has dry skin, but thinks his face and hair have not changed.

Previous medical history

- No tuberculosis, rheumatic fever, diabetes, kidney disease or epilepsy.

- Appendicectomy in childhood.

- Right inguinal hernia repair 1978.

Social history

- Mr Green initially planned an army career, but left the army to become a taxi-driver.

- He now has his own terraced house.

- His main hobby is building model railways.

- He gets little exercise.

- His diet consist of snacks during the day, with a high fat and sugar content and little fibre. He has a 'meat and two veg' evening meal.

- He smokes 20 cigarettes a day.

- He drinks two to three pints of beer a week at weekends.

Family history

Mr Green is married with six children. His uncle had an underactive thyroid, his father died from a heart attack aged 75 and his mother is well.

Drugs

- Aspirin, taken occasionally for headaches.
- Senna laxative, for the past four months only.

Allergies

- Penicillin causes rash.

Direct questions

- *Cardiovascular and respiratory system:*
  Smoker's cough producing clear sputum but no blood.
  Short of breath on hills, especially over the past six months.
  No chest pain, no palpitations.
  Mild ankle swelling, ?duration.

- *Gastrointestinal system:*
  Appetite normal, but weight rising.
  No nausea or vomiting.
  No indigestion or abdominal pain.
  Constipation as above.

- *Genito-urinary system:*
  No painful urination or frequency.
  No nocturnal urination.
  No blood.

- *Nervous system:*
  Vague headaches with no obvious precipitating or relieving factors apart from aspirin.
  No fits, faints or falls.
  Vision normal with glasses.
  Hearing normal.
  No pins and needles or numbness.
  No muscle weakness.

On examination

- Height 5 foot 10 inches (1.78 metres).
- Weight 13 stone 6 pounds (85.4 kg)
  (ideal weight 64–79 kg).

- Pale but not anaemic.
- Not cyanosed (blue), jaundiced (yellow).
- No xanthalesmata (fatty spots).
- Full face with puffy eyelids and watery eyes.
- Dry skin, normal hair and nails.
- Nicotine-stained fingers.
- Thyroid impalpable (not felt).

Cardiovascular system
- Pulse 60 beats/minute, regular rhythm.
- Blood pressure 130/88.
- No venous engorgement.
- Apex beat normal position (i.e. heart not enlarged), normal character.
- Heart sounds normal.
- Peripheral pulses full.
- Varicose veins both legs.
- Non-pitting oedema of both feet and ankles.

Respiratory system
- Intermittent cough with white sputum.
- Trachea central.
- Chest expansion normal.
- Percussion (tapping) note normal and equal.
- Breath sounds normal, with added wheezes.
- Chest resonance normal.

Abdomen
- Overweight.
- Appendicectomy and right inguinal hernia repair scars.
- Doughy.
- No enlargement of liver, spleen, kidneys.

- Normal bowel sounds.
- Rectal examination – normal.

Nervous system

- Cranial nerves normal, including hearing and vision.
- Retinae (back of eyes) normal.
- Power, tone, coordination and sensation normal in all limbs.
- Reflexes present, equal, slow-relaxing.

Diagnosis

Myxoedema.

The next section of the case notes would consider confirmatory investigations and health checks, followed by treatment and general health advice. These are considered in chapters 5 and 6.
What advice would you give Mr Green?

SUMMARY

- Doctors are taught to assess patients in a standardised way – your main symptoms, previous medical history, family and social history, medications, allergies, smoking, alcohol, diet, general questions, clinical examination.

- Clinical examination of someone with myxoedema may reveal slowness, cold dry skin, swelling, overweight, slow pulse and slowly relaxing tendon reflexes.

- There may be no convincing abnormalities on examination.

5

UNDERACTIVE THYROID – TESTS

In many cases the combination of some of the symptoms and signs detailed in Chapters 2 and 3 allow a doctor to make a confident diagnosis of myxoedema. But it is important to confirm the diagnosis by doing thyroid function tests.

LABORATORY TESTS FOR MYXOEDEMA

The doctor or phlebotomist (the person who takes your blood) will take a small sample of blood from a vein, label it carefully and send it, with an accompanying named card, to the laboratory. The laboratory will then spin down the blood in a centrifuge, separating the blood cells from the straw-coloured plasma they are normally suspended in. Other laboratories may allow the blood to clot and then use the clear serum. It is this plasma or serum that is then analysed in the various tests.

The thyroid function tests performed by different laboratories vary, both in the methods used and their specificity. It is therefore important for each doctor to know which tests his/her local laboratory use, and what the local normal ranges are.

Free hormone concentrations

The tests which are easiest to interpret are free T4 (thyroxine) and/or free T3 (tri-iodothyronine) along with TSH (thyroid stimulating hormone) assay. This means that, in most cases, the doctor does not have to allow for alterations in the levels of the carrier proteins associated with these hormones (see page 9). If the thyroid is unable to make thyroid hormones, the plasma concentrations, i.e. the concentrations of the hormones circulating in the bloodstream, will fall as the stores in the colloid in

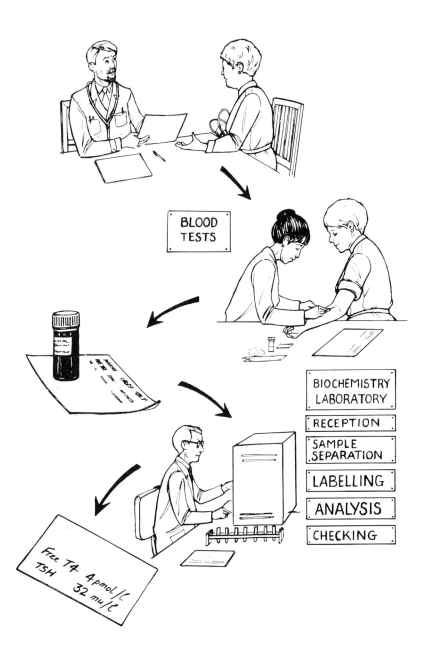

Testing for myxoedema.

the follicles (page 4) are depleted and not replenished. As the blood T3 and T4 concentrations fall the pituitary gland releases TSH – thyroid stimulating hormone – to encourage increased hormone production in the thyroid gland. This means that the plasma or serum TSH levels rise.

When John Green's blood was analysed by the laboratory his thyroid function tests looked like this:

- Free T4, 3 picomol/1.

- Free T3, 2 picomol/1.

- TSH, 45 milliunit/1.

Total thyroid hormone concentrations

Other laboratories use total T3 and T4 tests that measure the carrier protein levels as well. However, many factors can interfere with the interpretation of total thyroid hormone concentrations; one book lists over 40 drugs which interfere. Total T3 and T4 measurements may therefore produce confusing results, for example in women who are pregnant, who are on hormone replacement therapy or the contraceptive pill, or in people on some medications like the tranquilliser chlorpromazine. All these factors increase thyroxine-binding globulin concentrations and therefore raise the total T3 and T4 levels, which may in turn mask an underlying lack of thyroid hormone. Other drugs, like the anti-epileptic medication phenytoin, severe illness, major surgery and protein lack from any cause can all lower thyroxine-binding globulin levels and thus cause a low total T3 and T4, which may in turn produce an impression of thyroid hormone lack in someone whose thyroid is working normally.

However, the TSH measurement will provide the answer.

The production of thyroid stimulating hormone by the pituitary is not affected by carrier protein status, and will still be raised if the thyroid is not making sufficient T3 or T4. Some laboratories simply measure the TSH as their first test to determine whether someone's thyroid is underactive or not. But there is a catch.

Anthea Smythe also attended a thyroid clinic. These are her results:

- Free T4, 5 picomol/1.

- Free T3, 3 picomol/1.

- TSH, 0.06 milliunit/1.

Can you work out what the problem is? The answer is on page 52.

Borderline cases and the TRH test

Sometimes a person can have confusing symptoms and not wholly convincing signs of myxoedema. The blood tests may be a little uncertain as well. One way of resolving the problem is to wait a month or two and then see what happens; the situation will usually become more obvious on subsequent examination and tests. This is a practical course of action, for no doctor would wish to start what is probably life-long treatment without convincing evidence that it is needed. However, it may mean that the person who really is becoming hypothyroid feels below par for longer than necessary (see page 47 for further discussion).

A more satisfactory solution to the borderline problem is to see how the pituitary gland responds to stimulation. If concentrations of T3 and T4 are indeed lower than normal, then the pituitary gland will have responded by making and storing more TSH (thyroid stimulating hormone) than usual. If this is the case, an injection of TRH (thyrotrophin releasing hormone, normally made in the hypothalamus – see page 8) will then make the pituitary release its stores of TSH in a great whoosh, producing TSH levels of 20 milliunit/1 or more in men, 25 milliunit/1 or more in women, within 20 minutes after injection. In contrast the normal response shows a smaller rise than this. And if the pituitary gland is not working at all there will be no rise in TSH.

TRH may sometimes make people feel hot, and produce a tingling sensation in the genital area. This is a normal and harmless effect, but people with epilepsy should not be given TRH as it may cause a fit in people prone to this.

Thyroid antibodies

An antibody is a chemical produced by the white blood cells in response to any chemical trigger which the body perceives as a threat. Such chemical triggers are called antigens, and the antibody binds with the antigen and immobilises it. This is called an immune reaction; it is how we defend ourselves from infection. If you cannot produce antibodies you are at risk from infection – this is what happens in acquired immune deficiency syndrome (AIDS), and in some other conditions in which antibody production fails.

However, more frequently the opposite problem arises – unnecessary antibodies are produced. The body gets confused and starts to produce antibodies against a part of itself, i.e. it behaves as if one of its own chemicals is a threat. This process is called autoimmunity, and is nothing whatsoever to do with AIDS.

In thyroid disease the white blood cells make antibodies against parts of the thyroid gland. The autoantibodies that most laboratories measure are those that bind to microsomes – tiny particles inside the thyroid cells. These autoantibodies are called thyroid microsomal antibodies, while those against thyroglobulin (see pages 4–5) are called thyroglobulin antibodies.

The presence of thyroid microsomal or thyroglobulin antibodies does not in itself mean that you are hypothyroid, but it does provide supporting evidence, in conjunction with the clinical picture and other blood tests (see page 47).

OTHER TESTS

Blood count

About one in four people with an underactive thyroid develop anaemia – the body makes fewer blood cells because of the slowed metabolism. This resolves once the thyroid hormone levels return to normal.

Blood cholesterol concentration

One in two people in the United Kingdom has a blood cholesterol level which is above desirable limits. Myxoedema causes the cholesterol level to rise, probably because it is not cleared from the doby as efficiently as usual, although other chemical mechanisms contribute to the process. Before thyroid hormone concentrations could be assayed directly, doctors used to measure cholesterol to support the diagnosis of myxoedema.

Provided you do not have an underlying cholesterol problem, your cholesterol level will return to normal with thyroid replacement treatment.

Blood urea and electrolyte concentrations

Electrolytes are chemicals such as sodium and potassium, and are essential for normal body energy and fluid balance.

In myxoedema the blood sodium level may be low because less water is cleared from the body than normal, which in turn dilutes the sodium carried in the blood. Rarely the blood potassium may be high, although this occurs if you have adrenal insufficiency as well, the latter being an uncommon problem. Adrenal hormone lack can also lower the blood concentration of urea, one of the body's waste products.

Glucose

The blood glucose level will be normal in myxoedema. However, diabetes may occur in hypothyroid people (and vice versa), in which case the blood glucose will be raised. It is important to check this, as it will need treatment.

Electrocardiogram

This is an electrical recording of the heart's activity, often abbreviated to ECG (EKG in America). The tiny electrical signals produced by the heart as it beats are recorded by sensors placed on the chest and limbs. Usually the ECG simply shows a slow pulse, but it may also show other changes, suggesting that parts of the heart are not getting enough blood because their blood vessels are narrowed by fatty deposits.

SUMMARY

- The clinical diagnosis of myxoedema is confirmed by measuring the concentrations of thyroid hormones in the blood.

- Different laboratories use different assay methods and have different normal ranges.

- TRH will produce an exaggerated TSH response in myxoedema.

- The blood tests have to be interpreted in the light of the clinical picture and within the limitations of the tests.

6

UNDERACTIVE THYROID – TREATMENT

THYROID HORMONE REPLACEMENT

Just over 100 years ago Murray and his colleagues first showed that thyroid extract could cure myxoedema. Nowadays pure thyroxine is used, or, rarely, tri-iodothyronine. The dose of thyroxine ranges from 25 micrograms to 300 micrograms, 25 micrograms usually being too little to have much effect and few people needing as much as 300 micrograms. The standard maintenance dose is 100 to 150 micrograms once a day. Treatment is usually for life, but as thyroxine is simply a natural hormone which replaces what is missing it has no side effects, other than those of too large or too small a dose.

Starting thyroxine replacement
Thyroxine therapy should always be started gradually so that the body becomes used to it; too much thyroxine, too early, may speed up the metabolism too much. The usual starting dose of thyroxine is therefore 50 micrograms a day, increasing to 100 micrograms after two to four weeks and 150 micrograms after a further two to four weeks.

People with heart problems The speeding up of the body and the heart rate produced by thyroxine replacement causes an extra demand on the heart. In the few people with coronary atherosclerosis (furring-up of the blood vessels supplying oxygen and nutrients to the heart muscle) some areas of heart muscle may not get enough blood, which can worsen angina or cause a heart attack or coronary thrombosis. If you have had previous heart trouble, suffer from angina or have an abnormal ECG some doctors would start you on 25 micrograms of thyroxine a day for two to four weeks, under careful supervision often in hospital. They may increase your anti-angina treatment such as beta-blocker pills (like propranolol). Other doctors would admit you to hospital and start you on a small dose of tri-iodothyronine, changing to thyroxine later. The dose of thyroxine will then be increased very cautiously according to how you respond. If you have any chest pains after starting thyroxine treatment you must contact your doctor straight-away.

People with very severe myxoedema Occasionally people have such severe myxoedema that it slows down the functioning of other glands in the body, such as the adrenal glands. If your doctor is concerned that this may have happened he will give you steroid hormones (these are the hormones normally produced by the adrenals) to tide you over until the adrenal glands have recovered. Again, thyroxine treatment will be started very gradually, but in most cases, once the thyroid hormone levels are back to normal, the other glands return to normal too.

Maintenance thyroxine treatment

Once you are well established on treatment it is important to have just the right amount of thyroxine on a long-term basis. Too much and you will develop the features of thyroid over-activity. Too little and you will remain myxoedematous. But one of the problems in deciding the right dose is that different tissues in the body seem to recover from myxoedema at different rates. Furthermore, it may take six months or longer for the symptoms to resolve completely.

The best indicator of your thyroid status is you. How do you feel? Have your symptoms resolved? Or at least, have they improved? To back up your own impressions, your doctor can weigh you, measure your pulse rate, look at your facial appearance, your skin, the tissue swelling or myxoedema.

Thyroid function tests can help but should not be regarded as the sole indicator of treatment balance. The TSH level should have returned to within the normal range, as this reflects the thyroid hormone levels as 'perceived' by one tissue (the pituitary). The free T4 level itself should be close to the normal range, although this is less helpful than it might at first seem as it simply shows that the pills you are swallowing are being absorbed. The free T3 level might perhaps be more helpful as this is the active form of thyroid hormone, but is harder to measure for most laboratories. Your cholesterol will return to normal with adequate thyroxine treatment – unless you have an underlying cholesterol problem.

Tri-iodothyronine treatment

This treatment can be used in the very few people who cannot absorb thyroxine, or in people who can take nothing by mouth. It can be given by intramuscular or intravenous injection.

It is shorter-acting than thyroxine, a property which can in itself be useful in starting treatment in people with very severe myxoedema or heart trouble.

IODINE TREATMENT

Few people in Britain today have dietary iodine deficiency. In most areas of iodine deficiency people are now encouraged to use iodised salt. If you know your diet is iodine deficient you should discuss iodine supplements with your doctor.

Once someone has developed an underactive thyroid gland they need thyroxine replacement treatment. But do not be tempted to add to your doctor's thyroid treatment by buying herbal or health-shop remedies like kelp or other iodine-containing supplements merely because the label claims they are 'good for the thyroid'. (Some cough remedies also contain iodine, so check the label.) It is not a good idea to overdo your iodine intake as this has unpredictable effects (see page 50).

KEEPING HEALTHY GENERALLY

Obviously thyroxine replacement treatment is the most important factor in helping you to recover from your myx-oedema. But you must also keep yourself as healthy as possible generally to regain full fitness.

Diet

Although many people with myxoedema are overweight, this is mostly fluid and will disappear as the thyroxine treatment takes effect. However, if you were overweight before your thyroid gland slowed down, you will still need to do something about this problem. Because of the myxoedema your cholesterol level will also probably be high. This too will resolve, unless you have an underlying tendency to high cholesterol. However, while your body is sorting itself out under the thyroxine treatment, start looking at the sorts of foods you are eating, and their quantities. The constipation that often develops in myxoedematous people is another factor that you ought to consider.

Your diet is what you eat. A healthy diet should contain lots of high-fibre starchy carbohydrate foods such as wholemeal bread, potatoes in their jackets, beans, pulses and oat bran; but little sugary carbohydrate food like sweets, candies, chocolate, biscuits, cookies and plain sugar. Your diet should be especially low in animal fats like butter, cream, hard cheese or fatty meat. And if you were overweight before you became myxoedematous, do not eat too much as your appetite returns. If you are constipated eat plenty of soft fruit and vegetables.

Smoking

Smoking kills one in three smokers – it is so dangerous that you should stop immediately. Smoking is more addictive than heroin, so it can be very hard to give up your cigarettes. However, most people find it less hard to stop smoking altogether than to try to reduce gradually.

If your thyroid is underactive you are already at increased risk of coronary atherosclerosis – heart disease. And heart disease is a major risk of cigarette smoking; it is rare to see a non-smoker as a patient in a coronary care unit. So people who have an underactive thyroid gland should not smoke – it considerably increases your likelihood of having a heart attack.

Exercise

If your thyroid gland has been underactive for some time your muscles may well be weak and stiff, and they may ache. They will certainly take time to recover. To help them recover their tone and strength, discuss a gentle exercise programme with your doctor – it is very important to increase the exercise of each muscle gradually.

Skin and hair care

Your dry skin will improve as your thyroid hormone levels return to normal with treatment. However, it is helpful to reduce other causes of dry skin while this is happening.

Wear rubber gloves when washing up or doing other wet jobs, and avoid contact with detergents and other chemicals. Protect your skin from wind and sun. Moisturising creams may soothe itchy dryness, but it is probably better to use ones without strong perfumes that may irritate your skin. Baby oil in the bath or afterwards can also help, but be careful not to slip when getting in or out of the bath.

Conditioners may reduce some of the dryness in your hair. As the hair starts to grow again it may fall out alarmingly. This is because the new hairs are pushing the old ones out. Gradually, though, your hair will resume its previous thickness.

SUMMARY

- The treatment of myxoedema is thyroxine.

- Thyroxine treatment should be started with small doses, which are increased gradually according to response.

- Treatment is usually for life.

- Thyroxine is simply a replacement for a natural hormone, so its only effects are those of the natural hormone. There are no side effects if the correct replacement dose is used.

- Watch your diet – eat more fibre and starchy foods and less fat and sugar.

- If you smoke, STOP.

- Ask your doctor about a gentle, carefully graduated exercise programme to tone and strengthen your muscles and improve your stamina.

- Protect your skin from damage and use a non-irritant moisturising cream.

7

UNDERACTIVE THYROID – COMPLICATIONS

Most people with an underactive thyroid start to feel better within days of beginning thyroxine replacement treatment, and gradually continue to return to normal. This process may take several months, or occasionally years, depending on how severe the thyroid insufficiency was to start with. But a few people have problems, either with their treatment or because of their myxoedema itself.

PROBLEMS WITH TREATMENT

Undertreatment

If you are not taking enough thyroxine, your symptoms and signs of myxoedema will not resolve completely. If you still have any of your original symptoms after two months on the same dose of thyroxine, or if the symptoms disappear initially but then come back, contact your doctor. He can check you over generally and also send a blood sample to the laboratory to measure your TSH level and your free T4 or free T3.

If the TSH is still above normal or the free T4 or free T3 are low, you need a bigger dose of thyroxine. If, however, your thyroid hormone levels and TSH are normal, it may mean that your body is taking a long time to get used to normal thyroid hormone levels, or that the symptoms that are still troubling you are not actually due to myxoedema.

There is another problem with thyroid replacement treatment, though. Some people simply do not take their pills. It may seem very obvious, but if you do not take your thyroxine, it cannot cure your myxoedema. Thyroxine replacement therapy is not like a course of antibiotics – taken for a week and that's that. It is usually for the rest of your life – every day, every week, every month, every year. The occasional missed pill will not be a disaster, but a lot of missed pills will mean that you do not get the full benefit of your treatment.

Another cause of undertreatment (or overtreatment) is failure to understand the dosage of thyroxine, lack of communication or error. In Britain the pills come in 50 microgram and 100 microgram strengths. A microgram is a thousandth of a milligram. Some doctors may write the dose down as 0.1 milligram (mg) instead of 100 micrograms (0.1 milligrams and 100 micrograms are one and the same thing). This has led some patients to inform me that they are on 1 milligram a day, whereas others assure me that they are taking 'point oh one' daily. Some people even insist that the prescribed dose was 100 milligrams daily.

It is most important that you realise what strength pills you have and that you know how many pills you should take to make up your dose. Check the bottle each time you get a new supply from the pharmacist – is it the same dose as before? The dose ranges from 25 micrograms to 300 micrograms, but the vast majority of people end up on 100 or 150 micrograms a day; 100 micrograms is two 50-microgram pills or one 100-microgram pill.

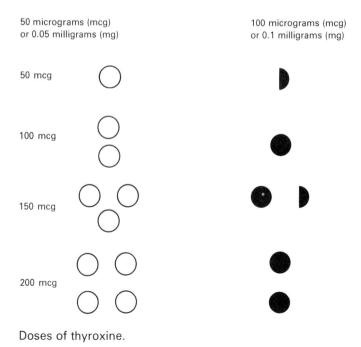

50 micrograms (mcg)   100 micrograms (mcg)
or 0.05 milligrams (mg)   or 0.1 milligrams (mg)

50 mcg

100 mcg

150 mcg

200 mcg

Doses of thyroxine.

Thyroxine is a once-a-day medication, and it is sensible to take it each morning when you wake up so that you do not forget it. I have met people taking it twice or even three times a day, in divided doses. It is a long-acting drug and it is not necessary to split the dose like this, although you will come to no harm if you do divide it up.

If there is any confusion in your mind, the most sensible idea is to take the bottle to the doctor or hospital or pharmacist every time. It's no use just showing them one pill, without the bottle – people keep doing this to me. But have you any idea how many types of little white pills there are?

Overtreatment

We all feel slightly unwell occasionally and anyone with a busy life feels tired sometimes. But if someone is feeling slightly unwell or complains of feeling tired, and they are known to have myxoedema, it is tempting for both patient and doctor to blame the symptoms on the thyroid problem. 'Let's increase the thyroxine', they say, 'that will improve things.' It may do, but only if the symptoms are actually due to a thyroid hormone lack.

Overtreatment, due to patient or prescriber error, is fortunately rare, but the examples above should alert you to this potential problem. Thyroid function blood tests will quickly demonstrate whether overtreatment is occurring. If the TSH is subnormal, the person is receiving too much thyroxine, which will be suppressing pituitary TSH release. High levels of free T4 in the blood also suggest this, although slightly raised free T4 is not uncommon in thyroxine therapy (it simply shows that the pills you are swallowing are being absorbed). A high level of free T3 – the active form – is more worrying, and suggests that the thyroxine dose should be reduced.

You may recognise overtreatment because it causes the symptoms of thyroid overactivity (see Chapter 9). There is some evidence which suggests that overtreatment increases thinning of the bones – osteoporosis. It is therefore important to avoid excess thyroxine. However, undertreatment may cause a rise in the blood cholesterol level, increasing the risk of coronary artery disease. A careful balance, avoiding either over-replacement or under-replacement, is, therefore, best although this is sometimes easier in theory than in practice.

COMPLICATIONS OF THYROID UNDERACTIVITY

Heart problems

Myxoedema can damage the heart in three ways:

- By encouraging furring-up of the arteries supplying oxygen and nutrients to the heart (coronary atherosclerosis).

- By weakening the heart muscle generally.

- By causing accumulation of fluid (effusions) in the bag which surrounds the heart (pericardium). This is called pericardial effusion.

The most common heart problem found in people with myxoedema is coronary atherosclerosis and its consequences. This occurs because of the increase in cholesterol circulating in the bloodstream associated with thyroid underactivity. It can cause angina (page 18) and, rarely, a heart attack or coronary thrombosis. If the myxoedema is treated and the cholesterol level returns to normal, the furring-up of the arteries may regress, although very long-standing hard lesions in the arteries may be permanent. Always tell your doctor if you have a pain in your chest. But remember, however, that most pains in the chest are not due to heart attacks.

Weakening of the heart muscle is called cardiomyopathy. It is debatable whether this is simply due to poor circulation or previous heart attacks from coronary atherosclerosis, or whether there is a separate myxoedematous cardiomyopathy, i.e. the weakening of the heart muscle is caused directly by the myxoedema. Both this and pericardial effusion can cause shortness of breath and pitting ankle swelling, i.e. the swelling pits if you prod it. See your doctor if you have either of these symptoms.

Hypothermia

People with myxoedema have a very slow rate of metabolism, and therefore find it difficult to keep warm. Rarely, elderly people – usually those whose thyroid insufficiency has not been diagnosed – are admitted to hospital with hypothermia. Hypothermia (hypo = low, thermia = heat) is a condition in which the person is unable to maintain their body temperature, so that they gradually cool down.

If you have an elderly relative with recently diagnosed myxoedema be especially careful to help them keep warm in cool weather. Once the thyroid hormone levels have returned to normal, though, they will respond to cold like anyone else of their age.

Myxoedema coma

This is now a rare complication of myxoedema and, again, is most likely in older people, especially if the condition is un-diagnosed, or is in the early stages of treatment.

If someone has very severe myxoedema or their condition is complicated by a major illness, the body metabolism may slow down so much that they become unconscious. They may become hypothermic as well. Myxoedema coma requires urgent treatment in hospital.

SUMMARY

- There are few complications of myxoedema.

- Undertreatment may be due to too small a dose of thyroxine, error or failure to take the pills regularly.

- Overtreatment may be due to increasing dosage for symptoms unrelated to myxoedema, or impatience as it takes time to return to normal.

- The commonest complication is coronary atherosclerosis and its consequences – this troubles few people and is treatable.

- Hypothermia and myxoedema coma are rare.

8

UNDERACTIVE THYROID – CAUSES

At some time or another everyone who becomes ill asks themselves the same question – 'Why me?'

Thyroid underactivity is common, especially in women, who
are affected about ten times more often than men. Two out of
every 100 women have myxoedema, and two in every 1,000
women will develop new myxoedema each year.

AUTOIMMUNE THYROID DISORDERS

Autoimmune conditions are those in which the body's own
(auto = self) defence mechanism, the immune system, attacks
part of the body, under the mistaken impression that it is
destroying a potentially harmful invader (see page 34). The
tendency for this to happen can be inherited, which is why
doctors ask for details of your family history.

Tissues which are particularly likely to be affected by an
autoimmune process are the thyroid, the pancreas (causing
diabetes), the stomach (preventing absorption of vitamin B12
and causing pernicious anaemia), the joints (causing rheuma-
toid arthritis) and the adrenal glands (causing Addison's disease
or adrenal insufficiency). If you have one autoimmune disorder
you are more likely than the population as a whole to have
others. The commonest such link is between diabetes and
thyroid disease; indeed, some doctors test all new patients with
diabetes for thyroid disease, and many test all new patients with
overactive or underactive thyroids for diabetes.

Some people with myxoedema inherit the tendency for
chemicals on or in their thyroid cells to act as antigens, i.e. to
provoke an autoimmune response; perhaps some outside event

activates these antigens, allowing them to trigger the body's defence mechanisms. The antigens are detected by white blood cells called lymphocytes. There are several sorts of lymphocyte circulating in the bloodstream, and some lymphocytes make antibodies targeted against various parts of the thyroid gland. Up to one in five people with myxoedema have antibodies which block the TSH receptors (see page 7) on the surface of thyroid cells. If these receptors are blocked the TSH produced by the pituitary cannot stimulate thyroid hormone production. Most of the antibodies which attack the thyroid can only be measured in research laboratories; however microsomal and thyroglobulin antibodies (page 34) are two which can be measured routinely.

In some cases the autoimmune response is such that lymphocytes swarm into the thyroid gland and produce antibodies that attack the thyroid cells and destroy them. In some forms of attack the thyroid tissue is replaced by lymphocytes, in others there are islands of normal follicles and islands of lymphocytes. Eventually, though, after a severe attack, the whole thyroid is destroyed and is replaced by inactive fibrous tissue like a scar.

This autoimmune thyroid inflammation with infiltration of lymphocytes is called Hashimoto's disease. It is often associated with a goitre and may occur without myxoedema.

The idea that thyroid underactivity is caused by one or a number of autoimmune responses is reasonable, but like so many ideas in biology, it may not be the whole story. For example, it is possible that the antibodies that we can measure are in fact produced as a result of some earlier attack on the thyroid, by a different mechanism. It is also becoming apparent that people with a tendency to autoimmune disorders may lack some protective mechanism against self-attack.

Premyxoedema or borderline myxoedema

Some doctors in north-east England measured thyroid antibodies in a cross-section of the population there. They found that between 2 and 4 per cent of men and 8 and 15 per cent of women had antibodies to thyroid tissue in their blood, thyroid antibodies being commonest in women over 40 years old; the average was about three out of every 100 men and eight out of every 100 women. They also found that about four in every 100 men, and 12 out of every 100 women had a raised TSH level. This suggested that thyroid underactivity was very much more common than was apparent from the numbers of people actually receiving treatment for it. If there are a lot of people with thyroid antibodies and a high TSH who have not felt ill enough to contact their doctors, should we be screening the whole population for myxoedema, all over the country?

Some centres have tried this. The problem is that when we actually find the people with thyroid antibodies and a high TSH, they may well have no symptoms at all and no abnormalities on examination. Furthermore, the free T3 and T4 levels in their bloodstream may be normal. We can do a TRH test (page 33), which often shows an exaggerated response, and this has led to the concept of premyxoedema.

Various groups of doctors and scientists have studied this problem. The north-eastern group (and others) found that, out of a hundred women with thyroid antibodies and high TSH, five will develop obvious thyroid underactivity each year. If we extend this calculation (which may not produce a completely accurate answer, for other factors are involved), by the end of 20 years all the women would have underactive thyroids.

There is debate as to the best management of this situation. One practical answer might be to measure cholesterol levels in the blood (see pages 34 and 37). If the TSH and cholesterol levels are both raised, this is evidence that at least two body systems are not 'seeing' enough thyroid hormone, i.e. there is not enough thyroid hormone circulating in the bloodstream to regulate the organs and cells responsible for producing TSH and cholesterol. The thyroid hormone should therefore be replaced until the TSH levels are back within the normal range. If the cholesterl fails to return to normal, despite the TSH having done so, the person probably has an underlying cholesterol problem unrelated to thyroid disease, and this will need separate treatment.

I should emphasise that this is just one person's view and that there are other, equally valid views on management. However, most doctors would agree that a person with raised TSH and thyroid antibodies should have regular checks to detect the onset of symptoms or signs of myxoedema or a fall in free T4.

TREATMENT FOR THYROID OVERACTIVITY

It is estimated that about one in three people with myxoedema have had surgical or radioiodine treatment for thyroid overactivity in the past.

Thyroid surgery

If you have had an operation to remove part of your thyroid gland in the past you are more likely than other people to develop thyroid underactivity later. The answer seems simple – there is not quite enough thyroid tissue to provide all the thyroid hormones you need. In fact it is a little more complicated, as most people who have had part of their thyroid removed have the operation to treat an overactive thyroid gland. People with thyroid overactivity may also have thyroglobulin and microsomal antibodies, which increase their likelihood of developing thyroid underactivity whether or not part of the thyroid gland is removed. About one in four to one in three people who have had a partial thryoidectomy (removal of part of the thyroid gland) become hypothyroid during the next ten years.

Radioactive iodine treatment
This is mainly used to treat thyroid overactivity. Radioactive iodine (also called radioiodine or I^{131} treatment, because that is the radioactive version of iodine used) carries a high risk of thyroid underactivity. About one in two people who receive radioiodine become hypothyroid in the ten years after the radioiodine was given.

Inflammation of the thyroid gland
Viruses can cause inflammation of the thyroid gland, just as they can cause inflammation elsewhere in the body. This is called thyroiditis (-itis = inflammation). There are several names for this condition – one version is called de Quervain's thyroiditis. Hashimoto's disease is a form of autoimmune thyroiditis.

Viral thyroiditis can cause painful and very tender swelling of the thyroid, the illness perhaps starting rather like an ordinary cough or cold. Initially, the inflamed follicles may release lots of T3 and T4 into the bloodstream and cause a temporary thyroid overactivity. Then the thyroid may become underactive until the inflammation has settled and the follicular cells have recovered.

Thyroiditis can be a temporary cause of thyroid insufficiency, requiring short-term treatment only. Hashimoto's thyroiditis (page 47) can cause long-term myxoedema.

Pregnancy
In, or immediately after, pregnancy the thyroid can temporarily slow down, causing transient myxoedema. Because it is transient it is important to follow the progress of myxoedema diagnosed around pregnancy very carefully, as some women will need thyroxine treatment for only a few months. In others the myxoedema is permanent.

49

IODINE

Iodine deficiency is the commonest cause of myxoedema throughout the world, and is mainly found in mountainous areas like the Himalayas, Andes and Alps.

Lack of iodine means that the thyroid gland cannot produce T4 and T3. This triggers the pituitary gland to produce TSH, but without iodine even TSH stimulation cannot increase T3 and T4 production. The thyroid swells as the numbers of cells inside it increase as a result of the TSH stimulation, and the person develops a goitre.

Iodine deficiency is no longer the main cause of myxoedema in the United Kingdom – iodised table salt is all that is needed to correct such a lack of dietary iodine in geographically deficient areas. However, you may still hear people talk about Derbyshire neck, describing the goitres previously common in this iodine-deficient area.

Iodine excess

Iodine has very complex effects on the thyroid. Large doses of iodine taken over a few days actually block thyroid hormone production by upsetting the balance of the chemical reactions which incorporate iodine into T3 and T4. This effect can be useful in the acute treatment of an overactive thyroid (see pages 74–5). If you eat too much iodine over a long time, for example from seaweed-derived remedies or from iodized cough sweets, this too can block the production of thyroid hormones in some people whose chemical pathways are not quite normal. These people can also develop thyroid swelling or goitre. In others excess iodine causes thyrotoxicosis (see page 87).

CONGENITAL MYXOEDEMA

This means thyroid underactivity you are born with, and it occurs in about one in 4,000 newborn babies. There are several causes, but the commonest is absence or abnormal development of the thyroid gland. Rarer causes include failures in the chemical sequence in which thyroid hormones are made.

PITUITARY GLAND PROBLEMS

All the causes of myxoedema described so far have been due to problems within the thyroid gland itself. But occasionally the thyroid factory can be capable of working well but be unable to produce the goods because of problems at the pituitary head office.

You will remember Anthea Smythe's laboratory results on page 33.

CASE HISTORY

Anthea Smythe was 41 years old when she went to see her doctor because she had had no periods for a year. Her periods had been regular until about three years ago, and it seemed rather early for the change of life. Milk had begun to leak from her breasts on occasions, even though she had not had a baby for ten years. Indeed, she had been sterilised, so she was certain she could not be pregnant now. She had also noticed that she felt the cold severely. Her muscles ached and seemed weak. She had started to feel dizzy when she stood up suddenly. Her husband thought she looked very pale.

On examination, Anthea's doctor noted that she did look pale and her skin seemed smooth. Her face was puffy, especially around the eye, and her pale cold hands and feet were puffy too. She seemed very weary, and admitted that she had been feeling tired and under the weather recently. Anthea had a pulse rate of 58 beats per minute (which is slow) and her blood pressure was 105/60 lying down, falling to 90/45 on standing, when she also felt dizzy. Milk could be expressed from both nipples, which were pale. She had very little underarm or pubic hair. Pelvic examination was normal. Neurological examination was normal, except for slow relaxation of her tendon reflexes.

If you look through Anthea's symptoms and signs, you will recognise some of the features of myxoedema. But not all of the findings can be explained by thyroid trouble alone. It is very rare for myxoedema to cause the breasts to make milk. One would not expect someone with myxoedema to lose their body hair. And although people with myxoedema can have a low blood pressure, severe postural hypotension (fall in blood pressure on standing) is unusual.

So her doctor tested her blood – her thyroid function tests were:

- Free T4 5 picomol/1.

- Free T3 3 picomol/1.

- TSH 0.06 milliunit/1.

Her thyroid was obviously underactive, as indicated by the low free T4 and free T3, but the TSH level was low too. That showed that the pituitary gland had been unable to respond to the low T3 and T4 levels – it showed, in fact, that the cause of the problem was not in the thyroid gland at all but in the pituitary gland. Further tests on Anthea's blood showed that levels of pituitary sex hormones were low, explaining her loss of body hair, and that Anthea was making insufficient steroid hormones, explaining why her blood pressure fell on standing. She was also making enormous quantities of the milk-producing hormone, prolactin.

A very special X-ray, a CT (computed tomography) scan, showed that there was a large tumour in her pituitary gland. The tumour was removed surgically through her nose and shown to be made of prolactin-producing cells. It was benign – it is exceedingly rare to find cancer in the pituitary gland – but it had squashed the cells making the pituitary hormones controlling sex hormone and adrenal steroid production, and also those making TSH.

Anthea Smythe had an uncommon but readily treatable problem. She is now completely well on full replacement treatment – thyroxine, steroids and sex hormones, the steroid hormones being started first so that her body could cope with the increase in her metabolism caused by the thyroxine. The only sign of the pituitary operation is a tiny scar on her lip. Looking back, Anthea thinks she had been feeling ill for at least three years.

HYPOTHALAMIC PROBLEMS

You will recall that the thyroid 'factory' is controlled by the pituitary 'head office', and that the pituitary is in turn controlled by the hypothalamus 'managing director' (see page 8) – it is the hypothalamus that makes TSH releasing hormone (TRH).

Extremely rarely problems in the hypothalamus, for example cysts, can cause a deficiency of TRH, so TSH is not made by the pituitary and hence T4 and T3 are not made by the thyroid.

SUMMARY

- Thyroid underactivity is common.

- The commonest cause of myxoedema in the United Kingdom is autoimmune thyroid disease. Many people have antibodies to thyroid tissue, but not all of them have myxoedema.

- Other causes are thyroid surgery and radioactive iodine, both usually originally used to treat an overactive thyroid gland.

- Worldwide iodine deficiency is the commonest cause of myxoedema. This can be corrected by everyone in iodine deficient areas using iodised salt.

- Sometimes too much iodine can cause myxoedema too.

- Temporary myxoedema may occur with inflammation of the thyroid, thyroiditis, and during or after pregnancy.

- Rarely, the pituitary gland stops making TSH, or, very rarely, the hypothalamus stops making TRH. This causes myxoedema too. There may be deficiencies in other hormones in this situation.

9

OVERACTIVE THYROID – SYMPTOMS

Other names for an overactive thyroid gland are hyperthyroidism (*hyper* means high) and thyrotoxicosis. It may also be called Graves' disease, although strictly speaking Graves' disease is the association of thyrotoxicosis, goitre and protruding eyes first described by Robert Graves in 1835.

As in Chapter 3 symptoms are listed according to the body system to which they relate.

How common are the symptoms of thyrotoxicosis?

Symptom	Percentage of people with thyrotoxicosis who have the symptom
Nervousness	99
Increased sweating	91
Oversensitive to heat	89
Palpitations	89
Fatigue	88
Weight loss	85
Fast heart	82
Shortness of breath	75
Weakness	70
Increased appetite	65
Eye complaints	54
Swelling of legs	35
Frequent bowel action	33
Loose motions	23
Loss of appetite	9
Constipation	4
Weight gain	2

GENERAL BEHAVIOUR

Anxiety and nervousness   Some people with an overactive thyroid feel as if their body is rushing out of control. You may feel as if things are going too fast for you, and you would very much like them to ease up. Some people simply have a vague feeling of anxiety or inner confusion. A few people feel so anxious that they go to their doctor for tranqillisers, 'to calm my nerves, doctor'.

Mood changes   You may find that you are euphoric, 'over the moon', one minute and in the depths of depression the next. You may find yourself snapping at people, irritable and knowing that you are being unreasonable but unable to stop yourself. On other occasions you may suddenly burst into tears over a minor problem, or apparently over nothing at all. Your family and friends may find this very difficult to cope with, and close personal relationships may suffer. These mood swings are due to the thyrotoxicosis, and are called emotional lability; they will settle as the thyroid hormone levels return to normal.

Overactivity   People with thyrotoxicosis can feel a compulsion to keep active, and may be completely unable to sit and rest. 'I always want to be on the go.' 'I can't bear sitting doing nothing.' 'I'm such a fidget, I just can't keep still.' You may clean around your family, or be always up and down re-arranging things or tidying. At work you may fidget or want to rush decisions. You can be a little difficult to keep up with.

Talkativeness   It may be your family and friends rather than you who first notice how talkative you've become. You may have so much to say, so quickly, that you cannot stop talking, and no one else can get a word in edgeways. Indeed, on one occasion, I was compelled to put a thermometer into a thyro-toxic person's mouth to keep them quiet for just long enough for me to listen to their heart.

Tiredness and exhaustion   The problem with thyrotoxicosis is that, although you are bursting with ideas and want to do every-thing yesterday, you may not have the stamina to carry it out. You may become tired easily and start jobs, only to discover that you cannot finish them. It is easy to become frustrated. In severe thyrotoxicosis you may become completely drained with the demands of your overactive metabolism, and become exhausted. Instead of burning to rush about all the time, all you want to do is sleep, and everything seems too great an effort. This is quite a worrying symptom in someone with thyrotoxicosis: firstly, it may not be immediately obvious that you have the condition, so that it may take longer to diagnose; and secondly, it means that your body is drained of energy and you are in urgent need of help (see page 82).

Skin, hair and nails Your skin may be thin, hot, pink and clammy. Women with thyrotoxicosis often complain of blushing very easily, the blush usually extending down the neck on to the top of the chest and lasting for some time. Your palms may be particularly red. Many of the symptoms of thyrotoxicosis mimic those of anxiety; anxiety also causes sweaty palms, but someone with thyrotoxicosis will find their hands sweaty all over.

Your nails may separate and accumulate dirt easily. Your hair may become very soft, fine, fly-away and difficult to control; you may find more of it in the comb or brush than usual, and notice some thinning out, although this symptom is more marked in myxoedema.

A swollen neck Many people with thyrotoxicosis will have a goitre, i.e. a swelling of the neck. Quite often it is just an appearance of fullness in the front of the neck, but if the thyroid swelling is larger necklaces or shirt collars may become tighter. Contrary to popular belief it is very unusual for goitres to cause pressure inside the neck, and swallowing and breathing are hardly ever affected.

HEART, CIRCULATION AND LUNGS

Heat intolerance If you have thyrotoxicosis, even in the coldest weather your overactive metabolism and vigorous circulation can make you feel hot. When everyone else is closing windows and putting on extra woollens, you are so hot you cannot bear it. You fling the bedclothes off at night, open the windows and turn the central heating down – your partner may not appreciate this at all. At work, you may still be in summer clothes while everyone else dons winter wear. You may also notice that your skin is very pink and feels hot to the touch, reflecting your vigorous circulation.

Increased sweating Many people with thyrotoxicosis also notice increased sweating; for example, you may find yourself

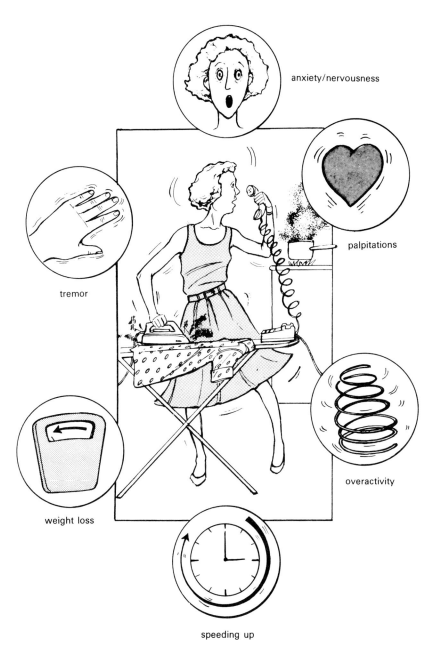

Symptoms of thyrotoxicosis.

sweating profusely after minor exertion. This, combined with feeling hot, may make you wonder if you have a fever.

Palpitations   As the increased thyroid hormones speed up the metabolism, the heart has to beat faster. You may become aware of this as an uncomfortable feeling or fluttering in your chest, especially at night, but also when you exercise. You may feel your heart pounding fast, usually in a regular rhythm, but sometimes erratically.

It is very helpful for your doctor to know whether the heart beats are evenly spaced (e.g. * * * * * *) or unevenly spaced (** * *** * * **) and, if possible, how fast your heart is beating during an episode of palpitation – try feeling your pulse (pages 101–2) and count the rate with your watch. Some people have intermittent palpitations – the heart starts beating fast when they have not been exercising at all. And rarely, the heart may go so fast that you feel faint or dizzy – your doctor needs to know about this.

Shortness of breath   This may be a part of your general lack of stamina – many people with thyrotoxicosis become puffed on hills, going upstairs or carrying heavy shopping. If you feel very breathless, especially while you are having palpitations, you should contact your doctor straightaway – he may need to give you some treatment to steady your heart.

DIGESTIVE SYSTEM

Increased appetite   You may start to feel hungry all the time. Second and even third helpings disappear quickly. You can start eating large snacks or have midnight feasts. Your friends look on enviously as you tuck into a huge helping of spaghetti bolognese – 'I don't know how you can eat all that and still stay slim.' But a few people, usually those with a very overactive thyroid, lose their appetite.

Weight loss   If your thyroid is overactive your metabolism speeds up and you start to burn-up first of all your fat stores and then, if the condition is not treated, your other body tissues. Even though your appetite increases, you lose weight, the weight loss sometimes being rapid. Occasionally, the increase in appetite is so great that people actually gain a little weight, but this is unusual.

Diarrhoea Different people mean different things when they talk about diarrhoea. For example, you may need to open your bowels more often than usual, but the motions are normally formed. Alternatively, you may also have loose or runny motions.

MUSCLES AND BONES

Shakiness Tremor or shakiness of the hands is a classical feature of thyrotoxicosis. It is present all the time, but is particularly obvious when you hold your hands outstretched. An artist with thyrotoxicosis found that drawing in fine detail was difficult because of this shaking. If you have to handle precision instruments you may have difficulties. The tremor is probably due to the increased sensitivity to adrenaline – the fright, flight and fight hormone – and is just like the shaking we all get when we are frightened or anxious.

Muscle weakness Although your thyrotoxicosis drives you to start a lot of energetic tasks, you may find that your muscles are too weak to achieve them. This weakness is often especially severe in the thighs and sometimes the upper arms; you may have difficulty getting up after squatting, or getting out of the bath. Because if affects the muscles closest to the trunk, it is called proximal myopathy. Sometimes your muscles may seem strong enough to start the job but tire easily. Your muscles may become thinner too – the medical term is muscle wasting.

Bones Prolonged thyrotoxicosis can also thin your bones, causing osteoporosis. This may produce aches and pains, particularly in the back.

SEX AND PERIODS

Irregular or absent periods Medical students tend to assume that thyroid overactivity is linked with frequent, heavy periods. In fact, the opposite is the case. Your periods may stop altogether, especially if you have lost a lot of weight. Someone who usually has regular periods may find them occurring at longer or shorter intervals, with little blood loss or just spotting. Your fertility may be reduced and there is a risk of having a miscarriage if you develop severe thyrotoxicosis in pregnancy.

Increased sexual drive   In both men and women libido may increase and you may want to increase your sexual activity. But thyrotoxic men may find intercourse tiring and uncomfortable because of their weak limb muscles, palpitations and shortness of breath.

EYES

Most people are aware of the link between fullness of the eyes and the thyroid gland. This condition, although very closely linked to thyrotoxicosis, is separate and is therefore considered in a separate chapter (pages 89–93).

SUMMARY

- An overactive thyroid gland is also called hyperthyroidism or thyrotoxicosis. Graves' disease is the combination of thyrotoxicosis, goitre and protruding eyes.

- General symptoms of thyroid overactivity include anxiety, nervousness, overactivity, talkativeness and tiredness.

- You may also feel heart palpitations, increased sweating and shortness of breath.

- Weight loss, despite increased appetite, and diarrhoea can occur.

- Other symptoms include shakiness, muscle weakness, menstrual and sexual problems.

- These symptoms resolve with treatment.

10

OVERACTIVE THYROID – WHAT THE DOCTOR LOOKS FOR

YOUR STORY

As with an underactive thyroid – indeed with all medical problems – it helps your doctor if you can list the symptoms which are troubling you most and if you can tell him as much as you can about them. How long have you had them? Have you ever had them before? What makes them better or worse? And so on.

Remember that no one has all the symptoms on the list, and some people do not notice any of them.

Previous medical history
Remember all your previous major illnesses and operations. Have you ever had a thyroid problem before? Do you have diabetes, Addison's disease or pernicious anaemia?

Family history
Do you have a family history of thyroid disease or of other autoimmune disorders (page 46)?

Your job and lifestyle
What are your work and home commitments? Are you coping with the demands of your overactive thyroid gland and your work? Is a young family wearing you out when you are already tired and weak with your thyrotoxicosis?

Eating, drinking and smoking   The caffeine in coffee and tea may add to your shakiness and speed up your heart rate if you drink too much. Alcohol causes flushing because it increases the circulation to your skin, and alcoholic drinks may add to your heat intolerance. And if you smoke, be honest about the number of cigarettes you get through a day. Then start working out how you are going to stop.

Drugs and medicines. Allergies   I have already discussed the drugs which may interfere with the older thyroid function tests (page 32). But some other drugs may mask your symptoms of thyrotoxicosis – the beta blockers (atenolol, metoprolol, propranolol) for example. Some people with thyrotoxicosis may be given tranquillisers before it becomes obvious that their problem is not their nerves but their thyroid gland; these too may modify some of your symptoms.

You must tell your doctor if you are allergic to any medication.

EXAMINATION – LOOKING FOR SIGNS

General behaviour and appearance   People with severe thyrotoxicosis may be so overactive that the air about them seems to quiver – I call this an agitated aura. With these patients the interview can sometimes be quite a problem for the doctor, particularly if the patient is very overactive and talkative. It is hard to get a word in edgeways and examining someone who cannot keep still can be challenging. One of the lessons I have learned is that the patient who gets the doctor feeling all worked up is probably thyrotoxic.

If you are thyrotoxic you are likely to be slim, with loose-fitting clothes. You may be wearing lightweight garments, even in cold weather, and will almost always have taken off your outer layers of clothing in the warmth of the hospital or health centre.

Hands   Your handshake will usually be very warm, and your skin may feel rather moist. Your rings may be loose. The palm of your hand may be red (palmar erythema). Your nails may separate from the nail bed at the tips, which makes them break easily and it can also be hard to clean dirt out from underneath. This condition is called onycholysis or Plummer's nails. Another nail condition is a swelling and increased curvature of the nail and end of the finger. These bulging nails are called thyroid acropachy, and is a condition that is not very common. If you hold your hands outstretched in front of you your fine

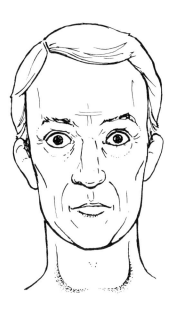

A person with thyrotoxicosis.

tremor will be obvious – especially if the doctor lays a piece of paper on top of your hands.

Skin and hair   Your skin is likely to be smooth, warm and pink and you may have the 'thyroid flush' from your face down onto your chest. This can linger blotchily on your chest for some time after the flush has ebbed from your face. (Some women blush like this normally.)

Some people with thyrotoxicosis develop areas of puffy thickening in their skin, especially on the lower legs. This is called pretibial myxoedema. Very occasionally it can become sore and purplish-red, so that it looks as if you have swollen ankles. You may have small patches of puffy thickening in other areas, and some people with thyrotoxicosis develop a thickening of the skin on the jaw line. Your hair may be thin and fine.

If you have an autoimmune thyroid disorder (see page 46) you may develop areas of pigment loss on the skin or in the hair. These white patches are called vitiligo in the skin and leucotrichia in the hair. They are simply a signal of autoimmune trouble and are not due to thyroid hormone problems. The white areas of skin burn easily and should be covered with sun block in hot sunshine. They can be camouflaged with makeup if their appearance troubles you.

Neck Many people with thyrotoxicosis have a goitre (see Chapter 9). Because the blood supply to the thyroid has increased your doctor may be able to hear the turbulent blood flow as a whooshing noise through his stethoscope. This noise is called a thyroid bruit.

Heart, circulation and lungs Your pulse will be fast (tachycardia) unless you are on beta blocker medication. Your heart rhythm may be irregular – called atrial fibrillation because the problem is due to an irregular quivering of the atria or upper heart chambers. Normally the area of nervous tissue in the heart that controls the beating of the heart – the heart pacemaker – sends out regular electrical stimuli that trigger contraction first of the atria and then of the lower, main pumping chambers of ventricles. But if the atria start producing fast erratic electrical triggers of their own, this irregular rhythm takes over and makes the ventricles pump at irregular intervals as well.

Your blood pressure may show a high systolic (pumping) pressure and a low diastolic (resting) pressure. This reflects your vigorous or hyperdynamic circulation.

Your heart, as heard through your doctor's stethoscope, will sound normal unless you have atrial fibrillation, in which case there will be erratic beats of varying loudness. Sometimes the doctor can hear the slight turbulence caused by vigorous blood flow and a murmur is present in systole (when the heart is pumping). This does not mean that the heart is malfunctioning, but simply that the blood is moving fast. If you have had severe thyrotoxicosis for a long time your heart may have become weakened, and you may have developed swollen ankles with pitting oedema (page 14).

There are unlikely to be any abnormalities in the lungs unless you smoke.

Abdomen Occasionally people with an overactive thyroid develop a swollen liver which can be felt under the ribs on the right of your abdomen. This will return to normal with treatment.

Eyes Your eyes may show some of the changes described in Chapter 15.

Nervous system Your tendon reflexes are likely to be very brisk – indeed the doctor may be able to elicit them simply by tapping your knees with his finger.

Muscles If you have lost a great deal of weight your muscles may be thin and generally weak. This particularly applies to the thighs. If your doctor asks you to squat down and then stand up without using your hands to help, you may not have the strength to do so.

CASE HISTORY OF THYROTOXICOSIS

Maria Stow is a 55-year-old art teacher in a college of further education. This is her case history, as written down by her doctor.

Patient complains of

- 'I'm losing weight.'

- 'I feel the heat very much.'

- 'My hands are shaky.'

History of presenting complaint

Mrs Stow has always had difficulty losing weight, but over the past two months has lost 2 stone (28 pounds or 12.7 kg), despite eating more than usual on holiday in Spain. Her appetite has increased and she wakes up hungry in the night and raids the fridge. She usually enjoys hot weather, but on this holiday was unable to tolerate it. She has turned the central heating down at home, and has had arguments with her husband as she keeps throwing the covers off the bed at night because she feels so hot and sweaty. They are now sleeping in separate beds. She teaches drawing and has been unable to draw fine lines because of increasing shakiness of her hands over this period.

On direct questioning Mrs Stow has also noted increasing fullness in her neck, although is unsure when this started, and sometimes experiences fast regular palpitations, especially on exercise. She used to open her bowels about every two days but now does so once or twice a day. The motions are normal in colour and consistency.

Previous medical history

- Fractured left leg ski-ing 1968.

- Pernicious anaemia 1977.

Social and family history
Married, husband an engineer.

- Three children, one married, two still at home.

- Lives in a four-bedroomed house.

- Non-smoker.

- Drinks about two bottles of wine a week.

- Diet mainly vegetarian, but eats dairy produce and fish.

Family history
- Her mother had diet-treated diabetes, while her maternal grandmother had goitre.

Drugs
- Vitamin B12 injections for pernicious anaemia.

- Occasional paracetamol for headache or back-ache.

- Temazepam in the past month for sleep.

Allergies
- None known.

Direct questions
- *Cardiovascular and respiratory system*:
  Short of breath on exertion.
  No cough or sputum.
  No chest pain.
  Palpitations as above.
  No ankle swelling.

- *Gastro-intestinal system*:
  Increased appetite.
  No nausea or vomiting.
  No indigestion or abdominal pain.

- *Genito-urinary system*:
  No pain or bleeding on urination.
  No increased frequency of urination.
  Menopause three years ago.
  No post-menopausal bleeding.

- *Nervous system*:
  Occasional headaches.

No fits, faints or falls.
Vision normal.
Hearing normal.
No paraesthesiae (tingling).

- *Musculoskeletal system*:
Muscles slightly weaker generally than usual.
Occasional backache for ten years at least.
Occasional pain in left leg since fracture.
No joint pains.

- *Endocrine system*:
No thirst, polydipsia (drinking a lot) or polyuria
(passing large volumes of urine).
No postural dizziness.

On examination

- Height 5 foot 7 inches (1.7 metres).

- Weight 7 stone 10 pounds (49 kg, ideal weight
53–67 kg).

- Overactive, talkative, grey-haired, blue-eyed
woman.

- Vitiligo on the arms and trunk.

- Warm, moist skin.

- Flushed.

- No anaemia.

- Fine tremor of outstretched hands.

- Bilateral exophthalmos (bulging eyes); lid lag
and lower lid retraction; full eye movements;
normal conjunctivae.

- Bilateral smooth thyroid enlargement; soft bruit
over right thyroid lobe.

Cardiovascular system

- Pulse 100 beats/minute, regular rhythm.

- Blood pressure 170/60.

- No venous engorgement.

- Heart not enlarged.

- Heart sounds normal; systolic flow murmur.

- Normal peripheral pulses.

- No ankle oedema.

Respiratory system

- Trachea central.

- Expansion normal.

- Percussion note and breath sounds normal.

Abdomen

- No masses or organ enlargement felt.

Nervous system

- Cranial nerves normal, including hearing and vision.

- Retinae normal.

- Power, tone, coordination and sensation normal in all limbs.

- Reflexes present, equal, very brisk.

Diagnosis

- Thyrotoxicosis.

- Treated pernicious anaemia.

The next section of the case notes would consider confirmatory investigations and health checks, followed by treatment and general health advice. These are considered in Chapters 11 and 12.

The causes behind Mrs Stow's thyrotoxicosis can be found on page 85.

SUMMARY

- Signs of thyrotoxicosis include agitation, talkativeness, overactivity, slimness and hand tremor.

- The skin may be warm, pink and sweaty.

- There is often thyroid swelling or goitre.

- The heart rate is usually rapid and the tendon reflexes are brisk.

11

OVERACTIVE THYROID – TESTS

THYROID FUNCTION TESTS

The measurement of T3 and T4 has already been discussed (see Chapter 5).

In thyrotoxicosis the free T3 and free T4 will be raised. The total T3 and total T4 will also be raised, but it is important to check that you are not taking any pills which will raise the carrier protein levels and give a false impression of thyrotoxicosis.

As the T3 and T4 levels in your blood rise, so your TSH produced by your pituitary will fall, and eventually its release will be switched off completely. These very low levels of TSH cannot be detected by some of the older TSH assays; however, increasingly, laboratories are using a highly sensitive assay system which can detect these tiny quantities of TSH. The TSH levels mentioned throughout this book assume that a highly sensitive assay has been used.

These are Mrs Stow's results, with normal range in brackets.

- Free T4 48 picomol/l (9–24 picomol/l).

- Free T3 17 picomol/l (5–10 picomol/l).

- TSH 0.02 milliunit/l (0.15–3.2 milliunit/l).

Extremely rarely, the pituitary gland develops a tumour which overproduces TSH, which in turn forces the thyroid to over-produce T3 and T4. In this case the T3, T4 and TSH levels would all be raised.

The TRH test
As in hypothyroidism (page 33), this test is used in borderline cases. If you have an overactive thyroid the pituitary will release very little TSH in response to stimulation by an injection of thyrotrophin releasing hormone (TRH). This flat response confirms the diagnosis.

Thyroid antibodies
Just as in hypothyroidism, the body may make antibodies to the thyroid gland – anti-microsomal and anti-thyroglobulin antibodies (see page 34). The other antibodies involved in the development of thyrotoxicosis cannot be measured routinely (see pages 85–7).

Thyroid scan
If you have one or more lumps in your thyroid, and in some other instances, your doctor will request an imaging scan of the thyroid. There are several ways of doing this.

The commonest scan in thyrotoxicosis is the radioactive iodine scan (this is not the same as having radioactive iodine treatment for your overactive thyroid). The scanning iodine is taken up most avidly by the parts of the thyroid that are most active in producing thyroid hormones. In this way the scan may show up a single overactive nodule which could then be removed surgically to cure the condition.

OTHER TESTS

Blood count
The white blood count may be lower than normal in some people with an overactive thyroid. Pernicious anaemia may co-exist with either hypothyroidism or thyrotoxicosis (as in Mrs Stow).

Liver function tests
While the thyroid is overactive the liver may temporarily malfunction. This liver damage can be detected by transiently raised blood levels of enzymes (special chemicals) normally retained in liver cells.

Blood proteins are also made in the liver, so their levels may fall if the liver is not working properly.

Blood calcium concentration

Up to one in five people with thyrotoxicosis have a raised blood calcium concentration (see page 83), the causes of which are complex.

Blood glucose concentration

Diabetes should be excluded in everyone with thyroid disease by measuring the blood glucose concentration. People with diabetes have high blood glucose levels.

Electrocardiogram

This is needed to check the heart rhythm, especially in atrial fibrillation.

SUMMARY

- In thyrotoxicosis blood concentrations of free T4 and free T3 are high.

- TSH levels are very low.

12

OVERACTIVE THYROID – TREATMENT

There are three ways of treating an overactive thyroid. Everyone will receive medication to start with. For many people this is sufficient to calm the thyroid and, over months or years, maintain normal function. However, it is possible to remove some of the overactive gland surgically. The third treatment is radioactive iodine.

Deciding on the best treatment for you is something for you and your doctor to consider, so what follows is a general guide only.

Children, young people and women of childbearing age usually only have anti-thyroid medication. Women over childbearing age, and men, often have radio-iodine treatment. If you have a single thyroid nodule producing too much thyroxine, a big goitre generally, severe thyrotoxicosis, or are having problems with anti-thyroid pills, then you may be offered thyroid surgery.

Some doctors believe that radio-iodine treatment should be more widely used. Others use anti-thyroid pills for many years. The important thing is that you and your doctor discuss which treatment is best and most acceptable for you and your thyroid.

ANTI-THYROID MEDICATION

There are three forms of medication which reduce thyroid hormone production – carbimazole, propylthiouracil and Lugol's iodine. Propranolol relieves symptoms of thyroid overactivity and may also have a direct effect on thyroid hormones.

Carbimazole

Carbimazole blocks the incorporation of iodine into thyroid hormone precursors and inhibits further steps in the chemical pathways in the thyroid. It also influences the autoimmune process and reduces antibody attack on the thyroid gland. In the body it is converted to the active drug, methimazole, and it is this form that is used in North America and elsewhere instead of carbimazole.

Carbimazole pills are usually 5 mg each. They are prescribed as a large starting dose, to achieve a rapid effect in controlling the thyroid, followed by a gradually decreasing dose according to response until a maintenance dose is reached. The maximum starting dose is 60 mg a day, but this is rarely needed and many doctors start with 30 mg a day. The dose is then reduced over four to eight weeks according to response, until a maintenance dose is reached – usually 5 to 15 mg daily. There is some discussion as to whether the dose should be taken all together once a day or divided up. The pills work equally well in most people either way. However, in severe thyrotoxicosis the pills should be taken every six hours, because of rapid metabolism.

Some doctors favour a block-and-replacement combination of carbimazole 15 mg three times a day and thyroxine 150 micrograms a day. This works on the principle of completely suppressing thyroid hormone production while preventing myxoedema with thyroxine treatment. This method of treatment usually needs less frequent follow-up than tailored carbimazole.

Contraindications   A contraindication is an indication that a given sort of treatment should not be used. In the case of carbimazole, the first contraindication is a previous adverse reaction to carbimazole. Breastfeeding mothers should not take carbimazole, and it should not be taken long-term by people with very large goitres or those who have goitres pressing on the trachea (or windpipe) – this is because the drug can cause the thyroid to swell even further.

Side effects   The most important side effect, which affects fewer than one in 100 people taking carbimazole, is that of lowering the white blood cell count. The white blood cells help to fight infection, the granulocytes by eating bacteria and the lymphocytes by making antibodies (page 34). If carbimazole reduces your granulocyte count it can render you liable to infections, particularly sore throats, (although it should be remembered that some people have a low white blood cell

73

count, due to thyrotoxicosis itself, before they start treatment – see page 70). If you develop a sore throat or mouth ulcers while taking carbimazole you must contact your doctor immediately so that he can treat it and check you blood count. Most doctors would advise you to stop your carbimazole until the blood result is known. Occasionally the platelets (particles which help blood clot) are low too. The blood count returns to normal once the carbimazole has been stopped.

Skin rashes, for example, itchy red spots, sometimes occur with carbimazole treatment, and settle once treatment is stopped. Sometimes they are so mild that it is not necessary to discontinue treatment. Some hair loss may also occur.

Other side effects are nausea, headaches, aching joints, swollen lymph glands and fever, and tingling and numbness.

Propylthiouracil

Like carbimazole, propylthiouracil inhibits the incorporation of iodine into thyroid hormones. It also blocks conversion of T4 to T3 in some tissues.

Propylthiouracil is usually made in 50 mg pills, the usual initial dose being 450 mg, either all taken at once or divided through the day. The dose will then be reduced according to response to a maintenance dose of 300 mg a day or less.

Contraindications Breastfeeding mothers should not take propylthiouracil, and it should be used with caution in people with poor kidney function. It should not be used in people with very large goitres or those who have goitres pressing on the trachea.

Side effects Side-effects occur in about three out of every 100 people who take it. They are the same as those of carbimazole, so it is important that you read the warning about low white cell count (page 73) carefully. A low white count is rarer in people taking propylthiouracil than those on carbimazole.

Lugol's iodine

This is only a temporary treatment – it is used before thyroid surgery and occasionally in very severe thyrotoxicosis. Lugol's iodine is a drink containing iodine and potassium iodide dissolved in water, the dose being 0.1 to 0.3 ml three times a day.

Contraindications Iodine therapy should be used with

caution in pregnant women and should not be given to breast-feeding mothers – it can cause goitres in their babies.

Side effects   Some people are allergic to iodine – you must tell your doctor if you are. Allergic reactions to iodine can include symptoms of a cold, headaches, watery or red eyes, sore throat, bronchitis, or skin rashes. Iodine is only given for a short course of treatment – long-term side effects include myxoedema, depression and impotence.

Propranolol

This is a beta-blocker – it blocks the effects of adrenaline (the fright, flight and fight hormone) on the heart, blood vessels, lungs and elsewhere. This means that propranolol calms the feeling of nervousness experienced by so many people with thyrotoxicosis, slows the heart rate down and steadies the over-activity. It may also limit the conversion of T4 into the active thyroid hormone T3.

Propranolol pills come in several strengths – 10 mg, 40 mg, 80 mg and 160 mg. This makes it especially important for you to know what dose you are taking. The usual dose in thyroid overactivity is 20 mg three times a day. Some people need more, however. The maximum dose of propranolol is 320 mg in 24 hours, but this much is rarely used in thyrotoxicosis and the more usual dosage range is 10–40 mg three to four times a day (a total of 40–160 mg in 24 hours). The dose will then be tailed off gradually as you start to feel better as a result of other anti-thyroid treatment.

Sometimes the doctor may start you on propranolol to relieve your symptoms while awaiting the result of diagnostic thyroid blood tests. Because propranolol improves your symptoms and signs of thyroid overactivity, you and your doctor can no longer rely on a clinical assessment as a guide to how over-active your thyroid gland is. You will thus have to rely mainly on the results of blood tests from now on.

Contraindications   People with asthma or a wheezy chest should never be given propranolol, as it may precipitate a severe or even fatal attack. It reduces circulation in the blood vessels to the arms and legs, and so should not be given to people with problems in these arteries. It also reduces the pumping power of the heart – harmless in people with normal hearts. However, if you have heart failure it may make it worse – except, in most instances, in thyrotoxicosis when it is used with caution, combined with other drugs.

Side effects A slow pulse, heart failure, wheezing, reduced circulation in arms and legs, aching muscles, lack of energy, sleep disturbance, bad dreams and gastrointestinal disturbances. People with insulin-treated diabetes may lose their warning of hypoglycaemia (a low blood glucose) if they take propranolol.

THE COURSE OF ANTI-THYROID TREATMENT

When a doctor first sees someone with thyrotoxicosis it is impossible for him to predict how long the thyroid will remain overactive and how likely it is to relapse, i.e. for it to become overactive again after it has returned to normal. Some people have very short episodes – a few weeks only. Others are thyrotoxic for months or years, and have several episodes. People with severe thyrotoxicosis and big goitres are more likely to relapse than those with milder disease and small glands. People with high levels of anti-microsomal antibodies (page 47) are more likely to become myxoedematous later than those with lower concentrations; and they may also be more likely to relapse into thyroid overactivity first.

After one year of carbimazole or propylthiouracil, three in five people have a further episode(s) of thyrotoxicosis, most of them within the next two years. Virtually all who are going to relapse do so within four years of stopping treatment. One practical management plan is to continue carbimazole or propylthiouracil treatment for two years and then follow the person regularly for the next four years. I personally use tailored doses of carbimazole for most people, with 'block-and-replace' treatment for those who show erratic swings of thyroid hormone levels in the early months of treatment, or those who have difficulty attending follow-up clinics.

RADIO-IODINE TREATMENT

This is a good option for most people over 45 years of age, and is increasingly being used in younger people nowadays. It is particularly appropriate for people who have had a lot of ups and downs in their thyroid hormone levels while on carbimazole or propylthiouracil treatment, or who have become thyrotoxic again after thyroid surgery. It is also useful for people who have difficulty taking pills or who have other illnesses.

The radioactive iodine is given as a drink or pills, and the iodine is taken up by the overactive thyroid cells; the radio-activity associated with the radio-iodine then destroys the cells that have absorbed it. As the cells are destroyed, so the output of thyroid hormones is reduced.

The dose of radioactivity is measured in milliCuries, and varies from centre to centre; some doctors first like to measure the uptake of ordinary iodine by the thyroid in order to calculate the dose of radio-iodine needed to return the thyroid function to normal but not cause myxoedema (thyroid under-activity). This is done less often now than previously, as it is still no guarantee that thyrotoxicosis will not recur nor that myxoedema will be prevented. Some doctors give a routine dose of 10 milliCuries, which is sufficient to control most patients' thyrotoxicosis but does not have a high risk of early myxoedema. However, some patients will need further doses.

Some doctors prefer to give a standard dose of 15 milliCuries to everyone, with the deliberate policy of causing myxoedema in most people. (Myxoedema is easier to treat than thyrotoxicosis, and will eventually occur in most of the people who have received radio-iodine anyway – see page 49). If thyrotoxicosis recurs, another dose of 15 milliCuries is given. This method has the advantage of ensuring that the thyroid is put out of action early in treatment so that thyrotoxicosis cannot recur. Because myxoedema is expected, the person is started on thyroxine treatment early on and does not develop myxoedema unexpectedly in years to come, perhaps in a situation when its onset might go unrecognised for some time.

Overactive thyroid glands will take up the radio-iodine avidly, where it gradually destroys the thyroid cells that have absorbed it. Thus the best effect, in terms of destruction of thyroid tissue, would be obtained in people with untreated thyrotoxicosis. However, it can be hazardous leaving someone with severe thyrotoxicosis untreated. Furthermore, as the thyroid cells are destroyed, they release large quantities of thyroid hormones into the circulation which can cause a thyroid crisis (page 82). Thus it is usual to control the situation by giving propranolol and carbimazole initially. The propranolol can be continued, but the carbimazole may be stopped a few days before the radio-iodine drink and then continued shortly afterwards until the radio-iodine has taken effect. It takes about six to ten weeks for this to happen.

Myxoedema Temporary or permanent myxoedema is common. If it has not been deliberately induced and treated in the early months after treatment, you should have yearly thyroid hormone measurements until you develop myxoedema. This may take 20 years or more.

Thyrotoxicosis and thyroid crisis The dose of radio-iodine may be insufficient to cure the thyroid overactivity and, as described above, there may be transient worsening of the thyrotoxicosis due to excessive hormone release.

Inflammation of the thyroid Occasionally the reaction caused by the radio-iodine inside the thyroid causes inflammation, and the gland may become swollen and sore, although this thyroiditis is usually temporary. The salivary glands occasionally become inflamed too.

Lumpy thyroid In later years the thyroid gland may develop nodules after radio-iodine treatment. However, radio-iodine does not cause thyroid cancer.

THYROID SURGERY

This is indicated for big goitres, especially the rare ones which press on the trachea or other neck structures; for people under 45 years old who keep having recurrences of thyrotoxicosis; and for young people who cannot take anti-thyroid pills for any reason. Some younger women will opt for surgical treatment because a medium-sized goitre worries them, or because they do not wish to take anti-thyroid pills. Planned pregnancy may be another reason.

As with all treatments of thyrotoxicosis there are many different opinions. Some doctors, especially surgeons, believe that all young people with an overactive thyroid should be offered surgical treatment. Others rarely use surgery. This variation in attitudes may reflect local expertise in thyroid surgery. Like all surgical procedures, someone who specialises in thyroid surgery may be expected to obtain better results than someone who rarely operates on the thyroid. There are so many areas of specialisation in surgery that one cannot expect every district to have a specialist in thyroid surgery.

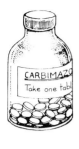 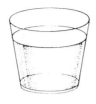 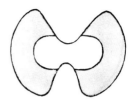

pills　　　　　　　radioactive iodine　　　　　　surgery

Treatment of thyrotoxicosis.

Preparation for operation

It is dangerous for anyone with thyrotoxicosis to have any operation unless the thyroid hormone levels have been returned to normal by treatment, otherwise surgery can precipitate a thyroid crisis. Before operation you need treatment with carbimazole or propylthiouracil and propranolol, probably for about two months, then for the last fortnight most surgeons would advise Lugol's iodine. This makes the thyroid easier to handle at operation, as well as reducing thyroid hormone levels.

Most surgeons would also insist on a detailed examination of your voice box to check the vocal cords. This is carried out by an ear, nose and throat specialist (otorhinolaryngologist), using a mirror to look down the back of your throat, and is done because about three people in 100 have a weak vocal cord without realising it, and the operation carries a very small risk of damaging the nerves which supply the vocal cords.

The operation itself – a partial thyroidectomy – requires a general anaesthetic, so the anaesthetist will check you before the operation. The operation then consists of the removal of about two-thirds of both lobes of the thyroid gland.

Winding down behind the thyroid is the recurrent laryngeal nerve – the nerve that goes to the vocal cords – which, as we have seen, can occasionally be damaged at operation. The other problem is that deep within the thyroid gland lie the four parathyroid glands which are responsible for organising calcium balance. The surgeon will search carefully for them so that they are left behind.

79

Problems of thyroid surgery

Myxoedema   About two out of 25 people who have thyroid surgery develop myxoedema (thyroid underactivity) in the years after surgery, those with high levels of thyroid microsomal antibodies being particularly at risk. Some surgeons remove most of the thyroid gland, aiming to produce myxoedema, and prescribe thyroxine routinely after operation. As with large doses of radio-iodine, this can be useful for people who have had very troublesome ups and downs of thyroid hormone levels over months or years of anti-thyroid treatment.

Recurrent thyrotoxicosis   This is uncommon but can occur, and occasionally nodules develop in the thyroid remnant.

Bleeding   Rarely a small blood vessel may bleed into the neck. This can create a painful blood clot, causing pressure on the windpipe, so it may have to be drained quickly.

Hoarse voice   Sometimes (in about three in 100 cases) the recurrent laryngeal nerve is bruised at operation, or becomes a little inflamed during the healing reaction after surgery. In this case the vocal cords do not work properly and you may become hoarse for a few weeks or several months. But it is very rare for the vocal cord to be permanently damaged.

Low blood calcium concentration   If the parathyroid glands have been bruised at operation, or their blood supply has been inadvertently reduced, they may temporarily stop working. This can lead to the blood calcium level falling dramatically, and can cause you to become weak, with cramping spasms in your hands. The cure is calcium pills or injections, followed by vitamin D pills. This situation usually resolves completely, as the parathyroid glands settle down after the operation. If it does not you will need long-term calcium supplements.

Wound problems   After the operation you will be left with a scar following a wrinkle line across your neck – ask the surgeon to show you where it will be before the operation. It usually fades until it is virtually indistinguishable from a wrinkle. Very rarely the scar becomes lumpy.

Other problems   All anaesthetics carry a very small risk of problems, and all operations carry small risks of damage to other local structures, of infection and of thrombosis.

Discuss all of the above, and any other worries you may have, with your surgeon. But you should always remember that the risk of problems is very small and the vast majority of people who have thyroid surgery have no complications.

SUMMARY

- The treatment of thyrotoxicosis is complex. Different patients need different treatments, and different doctors use different treatment regimens.

- Because thyrotoxicosis is a fluctuating condition, and because people's responses to treatment vary, the effects of treatment can be difficult to predict.

- Pills – carbimazole or propylthiouracil – suppress the production of thyroid hormone. Propranolol relieves the symptoms of thyrotoxicosis.

- Most people are treated with these pills at first or exclusively.

- Radioactive iodine destroys some of the overactive thyroid tissue. It is usually advised in older people.

- Surgery – partial thyroidectomy – which removes about two-thirds of the thyroid is another option, especially for large goitres.

- Radio-iodine and surgery may cause permanent myxoedema.

- All treatments may be followed by recurrent thyrotoxicosis.

- A person with an overactive thyroid needs regular medical follow-up for several years.

13

OVERACTIVE THYROID – COMPLICATIONS

EXHAUSTED THYROTOXICOSIS

Sometimes people with thyrotoxicosis are not overactive, talkative or nervous. Instead they lie in bed, exhausted, quiet, depressed and too weak to do much to look after themselves or their family. It is as if the constant stress on their body from the excess thyroid hormones has 'burnt them out'.

This is a potentially dangerous situation and requires treatment in hospital with carbimazole or propylthiouracil, and fluids and nutrients if necessary.

THYROID CRISIS

In a person with severe, untreated thyrotoxicosis or with inadequately treated thyrotoxicosis, a physical shock (such as an infection, an operation or an accident) or radio-iodine treatment can cause a thyroid crisis. This is when the excess thyroid hormones cause a high fever, a very fast pulse and collapse, sometimes with vomiting and dehydration. It is the body's response to the thyroid hormones rather than to the actual concentrations of T3 and T4 that is important. Another name for this condition is thyroid storm.

This uncommon and dangerous condition requires immediate hospital treatment to cool and rehydrate the person and control the thyrotoxicosis with large doses of carbimazole, Lugol's iodine and propranolol.

HIGH BLOOD CALCIUM LEVEL

About one in five people with thyrotoxicosis has a raised blood calcium level. If the level is very high it can cause vomiting, thirst and frequent urination, passing large volumes of urine (polyuria). The mechanism for the rise in blood calcium is complex, but the problem will settle as the T3 and T4 levels fall. Another reason for thirst and polyuria is diabetes.

HEART PROBLEMS

In older people the symptoms of thyroid overactivity can come on gradually, so it may be some time before the diagnosis is apparent. If the person has developed fast atrial fibrillation this may cause heart failure – shortness of breath, ankle swelling and weakness. The problem can be resolved with treatment for the overactive thyroid and the heart.

Palpitations
Sometimes people with thyrotoxicosis have intermittent fast atrial fibrillation – you feel very uncomfortable for a while, with an erratic pounding in your chest and occasionally feeling faint or short of breath.

If you have this feeling, try to count your heart rate and note the rhythm. Try to note what you were doing when the attack came on, as there may be little to find when the doctor examines you – these attacks rarely occur to order. Your doctor may arrange a 24-hour electrocardiogram; little sticky pads are applied to your chest, with fine wires leading to a small tape-recorder worn on a belt. This records every heartbeat for 24 hours, wherever you are.

These palpitations usually settle with control of the thyrotoxicosis.

THYROTOXICOSIS IN PREGNANCY

Pregnant women, or those who have just given birth, may develop a transient form of thyrotoxicosis, or occasionally myxoedema. Or women who are already receiving treatment for thyrotoxicosis may become pregnant. If the thyroid overactivity is not treated the baby may also become thyrotoxic (apart from there being an increased risk of miscarriage).

The usual treatment is anti-thyroid pills; surgery is very

83

rarely used, and radio-iodine never. It is very important to achieve normal thyroid hormone levels in the mother, but carbimazole and propylthiouracil cross the placenta, so if the mother is given so much of either of these drugs that she becomes hypothyroid, the baby will too and will develop a goitre. Some doctors give the smallest possible dose of carbimazole and see the mother very often; others give thyroxine supplements, to prevent the baby from becoming hypothyroid. However, it is unclear how much T3 or T4 cross the placenta into the baby.

What may affect the baby is thyroid stimulating immunoglobulin, an autoimmune antibody that switches on the hormone-producing activity in the mother's thyroid (see pages 85–6). Mothers with a previous history of thyrotoxicosis, probably with eye signs, may occasionally have a baby with a goitre and thyrotoxicosis at birth. It is therefore important to give enough carbimazole to suppress production of thyroid stimulating immunoglobulins when treating thyrotoxicosis in pregnancy.

Women who are receiving treatment for thyrotoxicosis should use effective barrier contraception until treatment has finished. If you wish to have a child and do not want to wait for perhaps two years of antithyroid treatment, there are two options. One is to have your child while taking your antithyroid pills. This does carry a small risk of thyrotoxicosis or, more likely, myxoedema to your baby, however careful you and your doctor are. The pregnancy will also involve a lot of visits to your obstetrician and endocrinologist. The other option is to have thyroid surgery, which will hopefully provide a definitive solution. Discuss the pros and cons with your doctor.

SUMMARY

- Serious complications of thyrotoxicosis – exhaustion and thyroid storm – are rare.

- High blood calcium levels occur in one in five people with thyrotoxicosis, most of whom have no symptoms of calcium excess.

- Heart problems are usually transient, but heart failure may occur in elderly people.

- Women with thyrotoxicosis can become pregnant and have healthy babies. They need careful supervision during pregnancy.

14

OVERACTIVE THYROID –
CAUSES

While most doctors agree that autoimmunity is responsible for most thyroid disease in the United Kingdom, whether over-activity or underactivity, there is considerable debate as to the precise sequence of events in both conditions. The situation is particularly complicated in thyrotoxicosis.

THYROID STIMULATING IMMUNOGLOBULINS

For many years scientists have known that people with thyro-toxicosis have chemicals in their blood which cause the thyroid gland to produce excessive thyroid hormones. Further work has identified an antibody called thyroid stimulating immunoglobu-lin (TSI) which can bind to the areas on the surface of thyroid cells usually reserved for thyroid stimulating hormone from the pituitary – the TSH receptors. Therefore TSI stimulates the thyroid to overwork, causing thyrotoxicosis. This form of thyroid overactivity can occur in a previously normal-sized thyroid gland or in one that has become enlarged, for example in an area of iodine deficiency.

A receptor is a place on the surface of a cell where a chemi-cal can link with that cell. It is rather like a keyhole waiting for a key. Several keys may fit into the keyhole, but usually only one turns the switch to make something happen. In this case the keyhole or TSH receptor is designed for the TSH key, but the TSI key not only fits the keyhole but turns the switch as well.

But why does the body make TSI? One theory is that the thyroid cells themselves are the cause of their own downfall. They may have slightly abnormal TSH receptors which trigger the production of the antibody, TSI, which then comes back

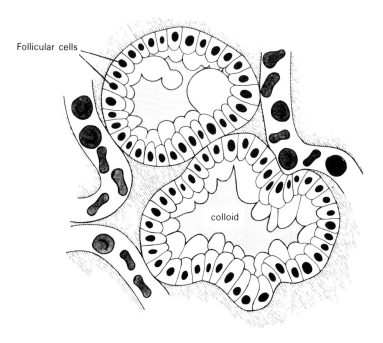

Follicular cells

colloid

Thyroid follicles as seen under the microscope in thyrotoxicosis. Note the depleted colloid stores.

and stimulates the overproduction of thyroid hormones. Another theory is (as with myxoedema) lack of protection against self attack; people with a tendency to autoimmune disorders inherit a flaw in their surveillance mechanism. Consider the immune mechanism as a security force in a large manufacturing plant; in the case of this particular flaw, either the security guards are asleep and fail to detect the production of TSI, the potential saboteur, or they are alert but carry guns without bullets and cannot shoot the saboteur down before it overstimulates the thyroid.

The techniques used to measure TSI and other constituents of this complex immune reaction are not available routinely in most hospital laboratories. However, it has been noted that people with high concentrations of thyroid stimulating anti-bodies often have high concentrations of anti-microsomal anti-body, and this can be used as a clue to what is happening. Other blocking antibodies, which stop the TSH receptor from working, may also be found in people with thyrotoxicosis; which is why you may spontaneously become myxoedematous. This tendency for thyroid conditions to swing from one extreme – thyrotoxicosis – to the other – myxoedema – makes it very difficult to predict what will happen to someone with thyroid trouble, and makes it hard to assess the effects of treatment.

THYROID NODULE

Sometimes a single lump in the thyroid, a thyroid nodule, may start to overproduce thyroid hormones. It is as if a small group of workers in the thyroid factory decide to work overtime, even though their product is surplus to requirements. In this situation the T3 may be high (and detected) before a rise in T4 occurs – T3 thyrotoxicosis. T3 thyrotoxicosis can also occur with other unusual thyroid lesions.

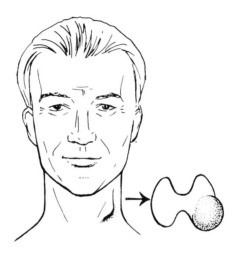

Thyroid nodule.

EXCESS IODINE

Too much iodine, for example in an attempt to correct dietary iodine deficiency, can switch on thyrotoxicosis in someone with an iodine-deficient goitre. This is called the Jod-Basedow phenomenon.

THYROIDITIS

Viral infections can cause thyroid inflammation, which may produce a temporary increase in the release of thyroid hormones from the damaged cells. The diagnosis of thyroiditis can be confirmed by a thyroid scan, which will show low activity in the thyroid gland because of the inflammation. This differentiates it from the more chronic condition of thyrotoxicosis, in which there is a high uptake reflecting the overactivity of the gland and its vigorous blood supply.

THYROXINE TREATMENT

People with myxoedema may sometimes take too much thyroxine, either because of an error or because they do not realise that the dose must be controlled carefully (see page 43). Alternatively, if someone with normal thyroid function takes thyroxine they may well develop the signs and symptoms of thyrotoxicosis, especially if they take it in large doses; this may occur if someone with borderline myxoedema is given inappropriate thyroxine. Some doctors also use thyroxine to shrink thyroid nodules, although this is unlikely to cause thyrotoxicosis as most doctors monitor thyroid function regularly in this situation.

People occasionally take thyroxine as a slimming aid. It must be emphasised here that the only use for thyroxine indicated in the *British National Formulary* is the treatment of thyroid disease.

TSH OVERPRODUCTION

Overproduction of TSH by the pituitary gland is a very rare cause of thyrotoxicosis indeed.

SUMMARY

• Thyroid overactivity is usually due to disturbances of the person's own immune system – autoimmunity.

• Thyroid nodules may produce excess thyroid hormone.

• Excess iodine can cause thyrotoxicosis in someone with an iodine-deficient goitre.

• Viral thyroiditis can cause temporary thyroid overactivity.

• Thyroxine overtreatment and TSH overproduction are rare causes of thyrotoxicosis.

15

THYROID EYE DISEASE

Many people know that people with thyrotoxicosis have prominent eyes and assume that the eye problem is caused by the
overactive thyroid. This is not the case; they are two conditions
that often coexist, and which have similar causes. However, it is
possible to have the eye problem with normal thyroid function,
an overactive thyroid or an underactive thyroid. In addition
thyroid disease does cause some changes, especially of the
eyelids.

About one in 20 people with thyrotoxicosis will have severe
eye problems. If the eye problems occur without thyroid
problems the condition is called ophthalmic Graves' disease.

SYMPTOMS AND SIGNS

The eyes may be watery and sore or gritty. They may be slightly
sticky in the morning. With severe eye problems they can
become very sore. You may notice that they seem very bright
and that they are bloodshot. Your vision may become blurred.

You, or more often your friends or family, may notice that
your eyes have become staring. Gradually the eyes may start to
protrude and you may discover that you have double vision.

Specific signs that your doctor will look out for are:

- *Bright eyes* Because of excess tear production or reduced
  drainage of tears, the eyes are a little watery and appear to
  gleam.

- *Blue eyes* People with autoimmune disorders are often, but
  not always, blue-eyed and develop grey hair early.

- *Red eyes* The white of the eye, or conjunctiva, may become
  bloodshot as the eye condition progresses. In severe cases

the redness may be marked and permanent, and there may be swelling of the conjunctiva, giving it a wrinkled appearance. The medical term for this is chemosis.

- *Puffy eyelids* This is especially prominent in myxoedema without other signs of thyroid eye disease. However, it often occurs in association with other eye problems, with fullness below the eyes, causing very obvious bags under the eyes and of the upper eye lid. The lids may be a little red, especially if you have been rubbing your eyes because they feel gritty.

- *Lid lag* Your doctor may ask you to look at his finger and to follow it upwards and then down in a big sweep. He is looking for a momentary slightly jerky lag of the upper eyelid as it follows the eyeball down. Normally the eyelid moves downward smoothly with the rest of the eye.

- *Lid retraction* This is what causes the staring appearance. The upper eyelid develops slight spasm which lifts it up, exposing the white of the eye above the coloured iris which lies under the invisible cornea through which we see. Normally the eyelids cover the top and bottom edge of the iris.

Exophthalmos

This must be the most misspelt word in the medical vocabulary. It means sticking-out eyes, and another name for it is proptosis.

To start with the eyes do not protrude very much, nor do they always protrude to the same extent. Sometimes just one eye may be affected – this happens more often in ophthalmic Graves' disease than in thyrotoxic Graves' disease, but the doctor has to exclude other causes of eye trouble.

The protrusion is due to oedema (fluid accumulation) in the tissues behind the eyes. The first sign may be apparent retraction of the lower eyelid, exposing the white of the eye below the iris. This is not true lid retraction, but rather the eye being pushed forwards. If the eye continues to protrude the eyelids may no longer meet over it. This means that the conjunctiva, or even the cornea, can get dry or damaged at night.

Ophthalmoplegia

The excess fluid behind the eye can enter the muscles which move the eye. As they become swollen they do not work so well. There are separate strap-like muscles to move the eye up and down and from side to side, and if just one muscle does not

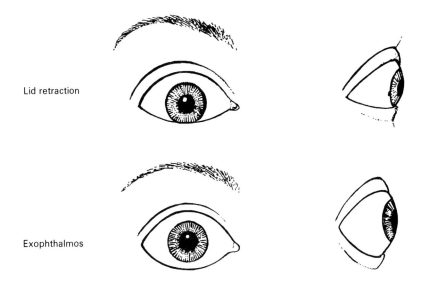

Lid retraction

Exophthalmos

Thyroid eye disorder.

work properly you will see double because the eyes cannot then be aligned properly.

The failure of eye muscle function is called ophthalmoplegia, and the double vision it causes is called diplopia.

Congestion

In severe cases pressure builds up behind the eye, the conjunctiva becomes red and swollen because the blood vessels draining the eye are being squeezed, and the cornea may be ulcerated because the eyelids cannot close.

As the pressure increases it presses on the optic nerve, which takes the visual signals from the eye to the brain for interpretation. This can cause visual loss. However, such severe damage is very uncommon nowadays.

DIAGNOSIS AND ASSESSMENT

Your doctor will obviously take a full story and examine you carefully. Your eyes will be checked in detail – what they look like, how well they move, and whether they protrude. The protrusion can be measured with a device called an exophthalmometer – a small frame with mirrors that is placed beside your eyes – while your visual acuity will be checked with a reading chart or an eye chart on the wall.

91

The doctor will also look at the back of the inside of the eye – the retina – with a magnifying torch called an ophthalmoscope. Sometimes eye drops are needed to dilate the pupil (the black part in the centre of the eye) to get a clear view of the retina; these drops may make your vision blurred for a while, but it will return to normal once they wear off. You may be referred to an ophthalmologist or eye specialist.

Obviously your doctor will check your thyroid function, and he may request scans or X-rays of your eyes or skull.

TREATMENT

Most people need no specific treatment for their eyes. The condition will follow its own course and usually settles eventually, although some people may always have rather fuller eyes than usual. Many endocrinologists believe that it is important to keep the thyroid hormone balance normal in someone with thyroid eye disease; marked overactivity or underactivity seem to worsen the eye condition. However, because the eye condition is separate, it may get worse after the thyroid has got better.

If the eyes feel dry and gritty, artificial tears (hypromellose) can sometimes make them more comfortable, although large quantities of artificial tears may be needed if you have severely protruding eyes. Double vision often improves as the thyroid hormone levels settle. If it persists an ophthalmologist can help with special glasses or prisms. If the diplopia does not improve surgery may correct the muscle problem. If the eye condition progresses and the surface of the eye and vision are at risk, steroid treatment (large doses of prednisolone) to reduce inflammation and to suppress the immune reaction, and azathioprine, which is an immuno-suppressant, may be effective. Sometimes very large doses of steroids need to be used first. Both these drugs have side effects, which you should discuss with your doctor.

Severe congestion can be relieved by surgically decompressing the space behind the eye. More minor surgery – sewing together the eyelids at the outer corner of the eye to improve closure – may also help.

You should remember, though, that most people have only minor eye problems, and that few need treatment.

CAUSES

As with the thyrotoxicosis itself, the eye problems seem to be due to the formation of antibodies to the tissues behind the eye and the eye muscles. There is debate as to exactly what happens, but the end result is the building-up of gel-like compounds behind the eye, with swelling of the muscles which move the eye. This causes the eye to bulge forwards and limits the movement of the muscles. Fluid accumulates in and around the eye. The process waxes and wanes on its own, making it difficult to evaluate different treatments.

SUMMARY

- Minor eye changes, for example puffy eyelids, can occur because of thyroid overactivity or thyroid underactivity. These changes resolve with treatment of the thyroid problem.

- A separate, sometimes more serious, eye problem can occur in people with thyroid disease (Graves' disease) or on its own (ophthalmic Graves' disease).

- In Graves' disease or ophthalmic Graves' disease there may be lid lag, lid retraction, and exophthalmos – eye protrusion. In more severe cases double vision or visual impairment may occur.

- In most cases the eye problems settle without medical intervention. In a few people, additional treatment is needed.

- It is important to keep the thyroid hormone levels normal in someone with thyroid eye disease.

16

GOITRE

A goitre is simply a swollen or enlarged thyroid gland; as the thyroid enlarges, for whatever reason, the neck fills out. But the swollen thyroid can also expand downwards behind the breast-bone or sternum – this is called a retrosternal goitre.

Teenage girls, young women and pregnant women may develop a slight fullness of the thyroid. This is completely harmless, and does not indicate thyroid disease.

SMOOTH SOFT GOITRE

This is the sort of goitre that accompanies thyrotoxicosis. It may simply be a suggestion of fullness in the neck or an obvious swelling on both sides of the trachea.

It is a very 'busy' goitre – you may be able to feel the blood rushing through as a vibration under your fingers, and your doctor may be able to hear the increased blood flow as a thyroid bruit (page 64). If you look at the thyroid tissue under a microscope, the follicular cells may be taller than usual and there may be holes in the colloid because it is turning over so fast. There are a lot of blood vessels.

A thyrotoxic goitre does not hurt and it is rarely big enough to cause problems because of pressure in the neck.

A MULTINODULAR GOITRE

This sort of goitre can arise for several reasons. It is lumpy and irregular, and some parts of it may be quite firm. It may be due to iodine deficiency, but is probably due to erratic overstimu-lation of thyroid tissue by TSH. Sometimes thyrotoxicosis can arise in a pre-existing nodular goitre.

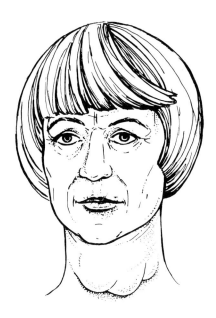

Multinodular goitre.

Multinodular goitres can grow large and may extend down behind the sternum. Occasionally they press on the trachea or gullet and limit breathing or swallowing; however, this is rare. What is more common is that once people have become aware of their goitre, they then start to feel discomfort in their neck, even though it is not actually pressing on anything.

If you have a bleed into one of the nodules it can suddenly swell up and be painful; a surgeon can usually drain this easily. If the goitre is large and its appearance upsets you, or if it is causing pressure effects, a surgeon can remove it (see pages 78–81).

SOLITARY THYROID NODULE

Sometimes a single part of the thyroid may start growing on its own. This is usually quite harmless, although occasionally solitary nodules overproduce thyroid hormones and cause thyrotoxicosis. However, it is sensible to check all solitary lumps in the thyroid by doing an ultrasound scan to see if they are cysts or solid lumps, and by doing an uptake scan using radio-iodine to see how active they are compared with the rest of the thyroid.

Thyroid cysts are virtually always harmless and can usually be drained as an outpatient procedure. But solid thyroid nodules that are not causing thyrotoxicosis need further investigation, one approach being to suck a minute sample out of the nodule with a fine needle. The sample is then studied under the microscope. However, because the sample is so small it requires special skills to interpret, and not all laboratories will have a pathologist with this specialist interest. The other approach is to ask a surgeon to remove the whole nodule anyway. This way it no longer troubles you, and the very small worry that it may be malignant is removed too. Thyroid cancer is rare and can usually be cured.

THYROIDITIS

In acute thyroiditis (inflammation of the thyroid) your thyroid may swell and become hot and tender, you may have a sore throat and tender lymph glands in your neck, and you may have transient thyrotoxicosis and, later, myxoedema. Your thyroid usually returns to normal, but occasionally it may remain swollen and firm although no longer tender. This may be called de Quervain's thyroiditis.

There is also a form of thyroiditis in which the thyroid becomes moderately swollen and very hard. Eventually you may become myxoedematous.

SUMMARY

- A goitre is a thyroid swelling. If you notice that your thyroid is swollen ask your doctor to check it.

- Girls, young women or pregnant women often have slightly swollen thyroid glands.

- A smooth soft symmetrical goitre is common in people with thyrotoxicosis.

- Multinodular goitres can become large and occasionally cause pressure effects.

- Solitary thyroid nodules can be cystic or solid. They need further investigation. The majority are harmless.

- Thyroid inflammation, thyroiditis, may cause painful thyroid swelling that settles.

17

LOOKING AFTER YOURSELF

If you have thyroid disease you can do a lot to help look after yourself. You can keep yourself generally fit, and can monitor your own condition – why wait until the next visit to the clinic before discovering that your thyroid has become overactive again? Why wait to learn that an increase in thyroxine is indicated? That is what this book is for, to help you to help yourself.

KEEPING FIT

To keep fit you need to eat and sleep well and exercise and relax regularly.

Your diet

The first thing to consider is your weight. Is it right for your height or are you too fat or too thin? If you are underweight because you have thyrotoxicosis, for example, you need to eat large amounts of healthy food to regain your proper weight. If you are overweight because you have myxoedema some of it will be fluid, and will disappear quite quickly with thyroxine treatment; but some of it may be fat, especially if you were overweight to start with. So watch the total amount you eat until the situation has become clear.

In a healthy diet, 50–60 per cent of calories should come from starchy high-fibre carbohydrate foods, and the rest protein and fat. Try to keep the fat content below 30 per cent of total calories. The sort of carbohydrates which are best are those which take a long time to digest, such as pulses and beans, wholemeal bread and pasta, brown rice, potatoes in their

Guidelines for body weight

Metric

Height without shoes (m)	Men Weight without clothes (kg) Acceptable average	Acceptable weight range	Obese	Women Weight without clothes (kg) Acceptable average	Acceptable weight range	Obese
1.45				46.0	42–53	64
1.48				46.5	42–54	65
1.50				47.0	43–55	66
1.52				48.5	44–57	68
1.54				49.5	44–58	70
1.56				50.4	45–58	70
1.58	55.8	51–64	77	51.3	46–59	71
1.60	57.6	52–65	78	52.6	48–61	73
1.62	58.6	53–66	79	54.0	49–62	74
1.64	59.6	54–67	80	55.4	50–64	77
1.66	60.6	55–69	83	56.8	51–65	78
1.68	61.7	56–71	85	58.1	52–66	79
1.70	63.5	58–73	88	60.0	53–67	80
1.72	65.0	59–74	89	61.3	55–69	83
1.74	66.5	60–75	90	62.6	56–70	84
1.76	68.0	62–77	92	64.0	58–72	86
1.78	69.4	64–79	95	65.3	59–74	89
1.80	71.0	65–80	96			
1.82	72.6	66–82	98			
1.84	74.2	67–84	101			
1.86	75.8	69–86	103			
1.88	77.6	71–88	106			
1.90	79.3	73–90	108			
1.92	81.0	75–93	112			

Non-metric

Height without shoes (ft.in)	Men Weight without clothes (lb) Acceptable average	Acceptable weight range	Obese	Women Weight without clothes (lb) Acceptable average	Acceptable weight range	Obese
4 10				102	92–119	143
4 11				104	94–122	146
5 0				107	96–125	150
5 1				110	99–128	154
5 2	123	112–141	169	113	102–131	156
5 3	127	115–144	173	116	105–134	161
5 4	130	118–148	178	120	108–138	166
5 5	133	121–152	182	123	111–142	170
5 6	136	124–156	187	128	114–146	175
5 7	140	128–161	193	132	118–150	180
5 8	145	132–166	199	136	122–154	185
5 9	149	136–170	204	140	126–158	190
5 10	153	140–174	209	144	130–163	196
5 11	158	144–179	215	148	134–168	202
6 0	162	148–184	221	152	138–173	208
6 1	166	152–189	227			
6 2	171	156–194	233			
6 3	176	160–199	239			
6 4	181	164–204	245			

jackets. Try not to eat much sugary carbohydrate food like biscuits, sweets, candies and cakes nor sugar itself.

The best sort of fat to eat is polyunsaturated fat or oils or monounsaturated oils like olive oil. Avoid animal fat like cream, meat fat, hard cheese and butter. Choose low-fat protein options like chicken, turkey, white fish or soya. It is especially important to have a low-fat diet if you have myxoedema.

If you have a poor appetite, make small attractive meals to tempt your palate. If you have a huge appetite try not to snack on chocolate or sweet biscuits, but choose healthier options. Eat plenty of fruit and vegetables, particularly if you are constipated because of myxoedema.

Alcohol

You can have alcoholic drinks, but in moderation. This means less than 21 units a week for men and less than 14 units a week for women. A unit of alcohol is half a pint of beer or lager, a glass of wine, or a single measure of spirits.

Smoking

This is extremely dangerous for your health, whether you have thyroid disease or not. One in three people who smoke will die from a smoking-related illness. However, if you have myxoedema you already have a high cholesterol level, which increases the risk of atherosclerosis (page 44). Smoking carries its own major risk of fat deposition in arteries, and therefore greatly increases the risk of heart or artery disease in people with myxoedema.

Stop smoking straightaway.

Exercise

It is always important to keep your body, heart and lungs in trim. However, one of the problems of thyroid disease is that you may not feel strong enough to exercise. Your muscles can be weakened by both overactivity and underactivity of the thyroid. They may ache, as may your joints. If the thyroid problem has affected your heart you may become breathless with exercise.

Whatever exercise programme you decide upon, it must be tailored to your individual fitness level, heart state and needs; it should be graded to prevent any undue strain on your body. This means that you must discuss your exercise plans with your doctor before you start.

Stress and relaxation

We live in a stressful world and many of us are exposed (or perhaps, more honestly, expose ourselves) to relentless pressures. Coping with stress as well as illness can be exhausting. It may delay your recovery.

Thyroid disorders may make you feel very unwell, and until the treatment has started to take effect you should reduce the external demands on you. It may be best to stop work for a few weeks. Women should enlist their families' help with the household chores; this is particularly important if your thyroid trouble has occurred with the arrival of a new baby. Try to relax, whether your thyroid is overactive or underactive.

People with myxoedema usually have no problem relaxing – their problem is getting themselves going. In contrast, people with thyrotoxicosis often find it very difficult to relax, the thyroid hormone excess pushes them on relentlessly. As your thyroid overactivity comes under control set aside a time each day to relax completely; try to sit comfortably, or lie down for the whole of your set time.

DECISION-MAKING

Because thyroid hormones affect the working of the whole body, they can affect the way you plan and decide things. Your memory may be poorer than usual. If your thyroid is overactive you may find it hard to concentrate on a single problem: if you are myxoedematous you may just fall asleep while you are thinking.

It is therefore important to realise that there may be a period of time – weeks or a month or so – when your mind is not as razor-sharp as you would wish. Things will improve rapidly as your treatment takes effect. However, while you are waiting to feel better, try to avoid decisions unless you cannot put them off. If you have to decide something right now, share the problem with someone you trust. Obviously some people experience more effects from thyroid hormone lack or excess than others – but be aware that you yourself may not be the best judge of your own decision-making capabilities while you are unwell.

MONITORING YOUR THYROID

It may help you and your doctor to keep a little diary of the progress of your thyroid condition. You may need treatment for ever if you have permanent myxoedema, or for many years if you have thyrotoxicosis. It can be difficult to recall what happened when, and which pills you took for how long. But if you have written notes of things you can measure, like your weight or pulse, as well as how you feel, you can see if your thyroid function is speeding up, slowing down or steady. But do not overdo this – keep things in perspective; a brief note of any events or changes and a few regular observations are all that is needed.

Weight
At the beginning measure your height and work out what weight range is acceptable for you (see page 98–9).

If you do not already have some bathroom scales, buy some and use them according to instructions – they should be on a flat even surface for best results. Make sure you know how to zero them. Get into the habit of weighing yourself regularly, say once a week or once a fortnight. It is best to choose the same time of day, with nothing on.

Pulse rate
The easiest pulse to measure is the one at your wrist – the radial pulse.

Hold your hand, palm up, and follow your thumb down to its base at the wrist crease. Two or three centimetres (about an inch) beyond this, in a groove between the tendons and the side of the wrist, is the radial pulse. Feel it lightly with the fingers of the other hand – it may take a few seconds to become obvious. Using a watch with a second hand count the number of beats for a minute. Count your pulse when you are resting in bed at night or on waking. The normal range varies depending on how fit you are, how rested you are and how anxious you are, in bed it should be between about 60 to 80 beats per minute.

You should be particularly interested in the trend of your heart rate. Is it getting faster or slower over succeeding months? Is it much the same? Count your pulse on the day when you weigh yourself and write it down. Note down whether the rhythm is regular (the beats feel like this * * * * * * *) or ir-regular (the beats may feel like this ** * * *** * **   *).

Neck circumference
Only measure this if you have a goitre. Use a tape measure and gently put it round your neck where it is widest, i.e. at the bulge of the goitre. Make sure hair, necklaces, etc. are out of the way. Note down the measurement about once a month.

General observations
- Has your face changed at all? Is it fatter or thinner? Is it pale?

- Are your eyelids swollen? Do you have lid retraction (page 90)? Look straight ahead and keep your eyelids relaxed to check. Are your eyes bulging? Are they bloodshot? Do you have double vision?

- Is your skin dry and cold, or hot and sweaty? Have you got patches of swollen or lumpy skin? Have you got a rash?

- Is your hair coarse, fine, difficult to handle, coming out?

- Are your nails brittle, a funny shape, hard to keep clean.

- Are your hands puffy or shaky?

- Are your ankles or feet puffy?

- Are your muscles weak? Can you stand up from squatting without using your hands?

Symptoms
One of the problems about encouraging people to take an interest in their bodies is that they suddenly have symptoms everywhere. Medical students and doctors are always mis-diagnosing serious diseases in themselves – it is an occupational hazard. Pulled chest muscles turn into heart attacks; a headache becomes a brain tumour.

I do not want to encourage you to worry over every minor symptom, but it is useful noting some of the more specific symptoms which might indicate that the thyroid gland is becoming overactive or underactive, or that it has returned to normal.

- *Temperature preference* Do you feel the heat or the cold more than other people around you?

- *Tiredness* Do you go to bed at the same time as everyone else, or earlier or later? Do you have to go to bed during the daytime (nightshift workers excluded)?

102

- *Chest pain* If you have any pain in your chest contact your doctor straightaway. But do not be frightened; remember that most chest pains are not heart attacks.

- *Palpitations* If you are unduly aware of your heart's action feel your pulse and note the rate and rhythm.

- *Appetite* Do you find it hard to clear one plateful, or do you ask for second helpings?

- *Bowels* Approximately how often do you open your bowels each day, or how many days are there between each motion? There is a wide range of normal bowel habits – you do not have to go every day. The main thing to notice is if there is any change from your usual bowel habit.

- *Periods* Premenopausal women should note down the date on which each period starts and finishes.

If you have any other symptoms note them down to discuss with your doctor – see the table on the next page. You do not have to have any symptoms – the aim is for you to be feeling fine.

Check-ups

The frequency of your medical checks will be organised by your doctor. In the United Kingdom you will be under the care of a general practitioner, who may investigate and treat you himself or who may refer you to an endocrinologist – a hormone specialist in a hospital. The specialist may continue to see you in his or her clinic, or may return you to your general practitioner.

Ask your doctor for the most exact results of your thyroid hormone tests and other investigations, and write them in your own record. Initially you may be seen at four to eight week intervals. Eventually you will be seen at longer intervals, perhaps annually. Long-term, I personally feel that anyone who is receiving treatment for myxoedema or who has ever had thyrotoxicosis should see his or her doctor annually. In most cases the general practitioner is happy to provide this follow up. If you are keeping an eye on yourself in between, you can ask for an early appointment at the first signs that your thyroid is misbehaving.

Thyroid check

Name: Iris Bloom
Diagnosis: Graves' disease (1.3.90)

Date	Weight	Pulse rate	Neck circ.	Treatment	Other drugs	Symptoms/signs	Other health problems
1.3.90	58 kg	120	34 cm	Carbimazole, 10 mg × 3/day Propranolol, 10 mg × 3/day		Sweaty, tired, palpitations, shaky, sore eyes	
14.3.90	59 kg	78		Same	Two aspirin for headache	Still tired, no palpitations eyes gritty	Pre-menstrual tension
28.3.90	60 kg	72	34 cm	Carbimazole, 10 mg × 3/day Stop propranolol		Less tired	
and so on							

SUMMARY

- You can do a lot to keep yourself healthy.
- Eat a low-fat diet and watch your weight.
- Relax and avoid stress and important decisions until you are well enough to deal with them.
- Exercise regularly according to your doctor's advice.
- Keep an eye on your condition. Note dates, test results and treatments.
- Note any symptoms, but do not frighten yourself by imagining things. If you are not sure whether you can feel something or not, it is probably not there.
- Attend your medical check-ups and ask your doctor about anything you do not understand.
- Look after yourself.

GLOSSARY

Medical words are defined within the context of this book. Some words may have other meanings in other contexts.

Addison's disease Condition due to failure of adrenal gland.

adrenal gland Gland found above the kidney which makes adrenaline and steroid hormones.

adrenaline (USA **epinephrine**) Flight, fright and fight hormone produced by the adrenal gland under stress.

allergy Abnormal sensitivity of the body to substances which are usually harmless. An allergic reaction usually produces unwanted symptoms.

anaemia (USA **anemia**) Lack of red blood cells.

angina Chest pain caused by insufficient blood supply to heart muscle (a form of ischaemic heart disease). Also known as angina pectoris.

ankle oedema (USA **edema**) Excess fluid in ankles, causing swelling.

antibody Chemical made by lymphocytes in response to an antigen.

antigen Chemical which triggers the body's defence mechanism and stimulates production of an antibody.

antimicrosomal antibody Antibody to tiny particles called microsomes in thyroid cells.

artery Vessel which carries blood from the heart to other parts of the body.

atherosclerosis Hardening and furring-up of the arteries.

atrial fibrillation Irregular quivering of the atria causing an irregular heartbeat.

atrium Upper chamber of the heart where the blood returning from the body collects. Plural = atria.

106

autoimmunity Condition in which chemicals normally found in the body act as antigens and stimulate antibody formation.

beta-blocker Drug which reduces high blood pressure, steadies the heart and prevents angina. All the names of beta-blockers end in -olol, e.g. atenolol.

blood pressure BP. Pressure at which blood circulates in the arteries.

bloodstream Blood flowing around the body contained within the blood vessels.

bradycardia Slow heartbeat, usually less than 60 beats per minute.

bruit Abnormal noise heard through stethoscope, usually due to turbulent flow in blood vessel.

calcium Electrolyte found in blood. Needed for bone strength, muscle function and other body functions.

carbimazole Drug used to reduce thyroid hormone production in thyrotoxicosis.

carbohydrate CHO. Sugary or starchy food that is digested in the gut to produce simple sugars like glucose. Carbohydrate foods include candy or sweets, cakes, biscuits, soda pop, bread, rice, pasta, oats, beans, lentils.

cardiac To do with the heart.

cardiac failure Reduced functioning of the heart causing shortness of breath or ankle swelling.

cardiomyopathy Disease of the heart muscle.

carpal tunnel syndrome Numbness in fingers caused by compression of the median nerve as it passes through the fibrous tunnel at the wrist (carpus).

carrier protein Protein circulating in the blood or other body fluids to which a hormone is linked during transport from the gland where it is made to the tissue(s) where it acts.

cells The tiny building blocks from which the human body is made. Cell constituents are contained within a membrane.

cerebellum Part of the brain responsible for balance and other coordinating functions.

chemosis Swelling of the conjunctiva.

cholesterol A fat which circulates in the blood and is obtained from fats in food.

cold intolerance Undue sensitivity to cold.

colloid Gel-like substance within the thyroid follicle where thyroid hormones are stored.

congenital Something you are born with.

conjunctiva The white of the eye and the inner eyelid.

connective tissue Inactive tissue which links other tissues.

constipation Infrequent and/or hard bowel motions.

coronary artery   Artery that supplies the heart muscle.
coronary thrombosis   Clot in an artery supplying heart muscle.
cretinism   Mental retardation due to congenital thyroid hormone deficiency.
cyanosis   Blue colouration, e.g. cyanosed lips. Usually indicates oxygen lack.
cyst   Hollow fluid-filled swelling.
de Quervain's thyroiditis   One type of inflammation of the thyroid gland.
Derbyshire neck   Goitre due to iodine deficiency found in people living in Derbyshire.
diabetes mellitus   Condition in which the blood glucose concentration is above normal causing passage of large amounts (diabetes = a siphon) of sweet urine (mellitus = sweet, like honey).
diarrhoea   (USA **diarrhea**)   Frequent and/or loose bowel motions.
diastolic blood pressure   Blood pressure between heartbeats.
diet   What you eat.
dietitian   Trained professional who promotes a healthy diet and recommends dietary treatments.
diplopia   Double vision.
effusion   An abnormal outpouring of fluid within a body cavity.
electrocardiogram   ECG (USA EKG) Recording of the electrical activity of the heart muscle as it contracts and relaxes.
electrolytes   Blood chemicals such as sodium and potassium.
endocrine   To do with the ductless glands (glands which deliver their hormones directly into the bloodstream). The thyroid is a ductless gland.
endocrinologist   Doctor specialising in hormone disorders.
epinephrine   see **adrenaline**.
epiphora   Watering eyes.
exophthalmometer   Device for measuring exophthalmos.
exophthalmos   Abnormal protrusion of eyes.
fat   Greasy or oily substance. Fatty foods include butter, margarine, cheese, cooking oil, fried foods.
fibre   (USA **fiber**)   Roughage in food. Found in beans, lentils, peas, bran, wholemeal flour, potatoes, etc.
follicle   Ball of cells within the thyroid where thyroid hormones are made. (Other meanings in other contexts.)
follicular cells   Cells out of which thyroid follicle is made, and that produce thyroid hormones.
free T3   See **free tri-iodothyronine**.

free T4   See **free thyroxine**.

free thyroxine   Thyroxine that is not bound to thyroxine-binding globulin in the bloodstream.

free tri-iodothyronine   Tri-iodothyronine that is not bound to thyroxine-binding globulin in the bloodstream.

gastrointestinal   To do with the stomach and intestines.

gland   Structure in the body that secretes chemicals.

glucose   A simple sugar obtained from carbohydrates in food. Glucose circulates in the bloodstream and provides energy.

goitre   (USA **goiter**)   Thyroid swelling.

granulocytes   White blood cells responsible for engulfing bacteria.

Graves' disease   Combination of thyrotoxicosis, exophthalmos and goitre described by Graves.

Hashimoto's disease   Autoimmune thyroiditis.

heart   Muscular organ that pumps blood around the body.

heart attack   General non-specific term for myocardial infarction or coronary thrombosis.

hormone   A chemical made in one part of the body and acting in another part of the body.

hydrocele   Fluid in the scrotum causing swelling.

hyper-   High, above normal.

hypertension   High blood pressure.

hyperthyroidism   Thyroid overactivity. High thyroid hormone concentrations.

hypo-   Low, below normal.

hypoglycaemia   Low blood glucose concentration.

hypotension   Low blood pressure.

hypothalamus   Part of the brain. It has several functions, one being production of thyrotrophin.

hypothermia   Low body temperature.

hypothyroidism   Thyroid underactivity. Low thyroid hormone concentrations.

impotence   Difficulty in obtaining or maintaining a penile erection.

incoordination   Lack of coordination.

infarction   Condition in which a body tissue dies from lack of blood supply – irreversible.

iodine   Chemical required for thyroid hormone manufacture.

iodine 131 or I^{131}   Radioactive iodine used to treat thyrotoxicosis.

iris   Coloured part of eye forming the ring which contracts or expands around the central pupil.

ischaemia   Condition in which a body tissue has insufficient blood supply – reversible.

ischaemic heart disease   An illness in which the blood supply to the heart muscle is insufficient.

isthmus   Narrow neck of tissue connecting the left and right lobes of the thyroid.

jaundice   Yellow colouration due to bile pigments.

Jod-Basedow phenomenon   Hyperthyroidism induced by iodine in someone who was previously iodine-deficient.

kilocalories   Cals or kcals. A measure of energy, for example in food or used up in exercise.

kilojoules   Another measure of energy. One kilocalorie = 4.2 kilojoules.

larynx   Voice box.

left ventricle   Chamber of the heart which pumps oxygenated blood into the aorta.

left ventricular failure   Reduced functioning of the left pumping chamber of the heart causing fluid to build up in the lungs and shortness of breath.

leuconychia   White nails.

leucotrichia   White hair.

libido   Sexual urge.

lid lag   Slow descent of upper eyelid and downward gaze in someone with thyroid eye disease.

lid retraction   apparent drawing back of upper eyelid to show white of eye above iris in someone with thyroid eye disease.

lipid   General name for fats found in the body.

liver   Large organ in upper right abdomen that acts as energy store, chemical factory and detoxifying unit, and that produces bile.

lobe   Part of thyroid.

Lugol's iodine   Iodine preparation used in the treatment of thyrotoxicosis.

lymphocyte   White blood cell that produces antibodies in response to an antigen.

malaise   Feeling vaguely unwell or uncomfortable.

median nerve   Nerve that supplies part of the hand.

metabolism   The chemical processing of substances in the body.

microgram (=μ)   One-millionth of a gram; one-thousandth of a milligram. Measure of weight.

milligram (mg)   One-thousandth of a gram. Measure of weight.

millimol per litre (mmol/l)   Measure of concentration of substances in the blood.

mitochondria   Tiny structures in which many chemical reactions occur. They are found inside cells.

multinodular goitre   Thyroid swelling with lots of lumps in it.
muscle wasting   Loss of muscle bulk.
myocardial infarction   Death of heart muscle caused by lack of blood supply.
myocardium   Heart muscle.
myopathy   Muscle disorder.
myxoedema   Thyroid underactivity or hypothyroidism in which there is swelling which does not indent with finger pressure.
nerve   Cable carrying signals to or from the brain and spinal cord.
neuroelectrophysiology   Study of the way nerves work.
neuropathy   Abnormality of the nerves.
nodule   Single lump.
nutritionist   Trained professional who studies diets. Nutritionists may be dietitians, and vice versa.
obese   Overweight, fat.
obesity   Condition of being overweight or fat.
oedema   (USA *edema*)   Swelling.
onycholysis   Condition in which fingernails separate from the nail bed and break easily.
ophthalmic   To do with the eye.
ophthalmic Graves' disease   Eye protrusion without abnormal thyroid function.
ophthalmologist   Doctor specialising in eye disorders.
ophthalmoplegia   Paralysis of eye muscle. Usually causes double vision.
ophthalmoscope   Magnifying torch with which the doctor looks into your eyes.
oral   Taken by mouth.
osteoporosis   Thinning of the bones.
palpitations   Awareness of irregular or abnormally fast heartbeat.
paraesthesiae   Pins and needles or tingling.
partial thyroidectomy   Partial surgical removal of the thyroid gland.
-pathy   Disease or abnormality, e.g. neuropathy, retinopathy.
Pendred's syndrome   Rare inherited disorder with myxoedema, deafness and white hair.
pericardial effusion   Fluid within the pericardium.
pericardium   Membranous bag within which the heart beats.
pernicious anaemia   Anaemia due to vitamin B12 deficiency.
phlebotomist   Person who takes blood samples.
picomol per litre (pmol/l)   A micromicromol or a thousand-millionth of a millimol. Unit of concentration of substances in the blood.

pituitary Gland in head that controls the function of most other endocrine glands.

pituitary stalk Thin stem of tissue connecting the pituitary gland to the hypothalamus.

plasma Clear fluid in which the red blood cells are suspended. It is separated off by centrifuging unclotted blood.

platelets Particles found in the bloodstream which are essential for blood clotting.

Plummer's nails Onycholysis.

polydipsia Drinking large volumes of fluid.

polyunsaturated fats Fats containing vegetable oils such as sunflower seed oil.

polyuria Passing large volumes of urine frequently.

postural hypotension Fall in blood pressure on standing.

potassium Essential blood chemical.

premyxoedema State that precedes myxoedema – TSH is raised and thyroid antibodies are present, but thyroid hormone levels are normal.

pretibial myxoedema Thickening or swelling of the skin, usually over the lower leg, in people with thyroid hormone abnormalities.

prolactin Milk-producing hormone made in the pituitary.

propranolol Beta-blocker drug used to relieve the symptoms of thyrotoxicosis.

propylthiouracil Drug that reduces the production of thyroid hormones. Used in the treatment of thyrotoxicosis.

protein Dietary constituent required for body growth and repair. Found in meat and cheese, for example.

proximal myopathy Myopathy or muscle disorder of the limb muscles closest to the trunk.

radioactive iodine Form of iodine that is radioactive. Used to treat thyrotoxicosis.

radioiodine Radioactive iodine.

receptor Place on the cell wall with which a chemical or hormone links.

rectal To do with the rectum.

rectum Back passage, which holds faeces just before they are passed.

recurrent laryngeal nerve Nerve that controls vocal cords in the larynx.

reflex Involuntary action.

renal To do with the kidney.

retina Light sensitive tissue at the back of the eye.

retrosternal goitre Goitre that extends down behind the sternum or breastbone.

saturated fats   Fats usually found in animal products such as those in dairy products, meat fat. Also in coconut and some other plants.

secrete   Actively release a chemical, e.g. a hormone, into the circulation.

serum   Clear fluid obtained when blood clots. On clotting some components of plasma are bound up in the blood clot. Thus serum is different from plasma.

sign   something you can see, touch, smell or hear.

sodium   Essential blood chemical.

sternum   Breastbone.

steroid hormone   A hormone produced by the adrenal gland.

subcutaneous   The fatty tissues under the skin.

symptom   Something a person experiences.

systolic blood pressure   Pumping pressure.

T3   Abreviation for tri-iodothyronine.

T4   Abbreviation for thyroxine.

tachycardia   Unduly fast heart rate.

TBG   Thyroxine-binding globulin.

tendon reflex   Involuntary muscle contraction on tapping a tendon.

testosterone   Male sex hormone.

thrombosis   Clotting of blood.

thrombus   A blood clot.

thyroglobulin   Chemical to which T4 and T3 are bound during storage within the thyroid follicle in the thyroid gland.

thyroglobulin antibodies   Antibodies targeted against thyroglobulin as an antigen.

thyroid   Endocrine gland in neck.

thyroid acropachy   Increased curvature of nails, found in association with thyrotoxicosis.

thyroid antibodies   Antibodies targeted against antigens that form part of the thyroid gland.

thyroid bruit   Noise heard through stethoscope due to blood flowing through engorged thyroid gland.

thyroid crisis   State of collapse due to severe thyrotoxicosis.

thyroidectomy   Surgical removal of thyroid gland.

thyroiditis   Inflammation of the thyroid gland.

thyroid nodule   Lump in thyroid. May be solid or fluid-filled.

thyroid-stimulating hormone   Thyrotrophin or TSH. Made in the pituitary, it stimulates T3 and T4 production by the thyroid gland.

thyroid-stimulating immunoglobulin (TSI)   Chemical that acts like TSH in stimulating thyroid hormone production.

thyroid storm   Thyroid crisis.

thyrotoxicosis Thyroid overactivity or hyperthyroidism. Originally associated with severe illness, i.e. 'toxicosis', but now more generally used.

thyrotrophin Thyroid-stimulating hormone (TSH) made in the pituitary gland.

thyrotrophin-releasing hormone TRH Made in the hypo-thalamus, it stimulates production of TSH by the pituitary.

thyroxine (T4) Hormone containing four iodine units made by the thyroid gland.

thyroxine-binding globulin Protein which carries thyroxine in the blood.

total T3 T3 or tri-iodothyronine bound to its carrier protein.

total T4 T4 or thyroxine bound to its carrier protein.

trachea Windpipe.

TRH Abbreviation for thyrotrophin-releasing hormone or TSH-releasing hormone.

triglyceride Form of fat that circulates in the bloodstream.

tri-iodothyronine (T3) Hormone containing three iodine units made by the thyroid gland and produced in some tissues from thyroxine. The active thyroid hormone.

TSH Abbreviation for thyroid-stimulating hormone.

TSI Thyroid-stimulating immunuglobulin.

ultrasound scan Scan of a part of the body using sound waves.

urea Blood chemical; waste substance excreted in urine.

ventricle Pumping chamber of heart.

visual acuity Sharpness of vision.

vitiligo Areas of white depigmented skin.

vocal cord Flap of muscle in larynx or voice box. Blowing air out past the variable closing and opening of the two vocal cords allows speech and singing.

xanthelamsa Fatty plaque above or below eye.

xanthoma Fatty lump in skin or tendon.

INDEX

Page numbers in *italic* refer to the illustrations

115